Palliative Care in Neurological Disease

pital

Palliative Care in Neurological Disease

A TEAM APPROACH

Edited by

JUDI BYRNE

End of Life and Bereavement Care Lead
Sue Ryder Care Central Office, London

PENNY McNAMARA

Consultant in Palliative Medicine
Sue Ryder Care
St John's Hospice, Moggerhanger, Bedfordshire

JANE SEYMOUR

Sue Ryder Care Professor in Palliative and End of Life Studies
School of Nursing, Midwifery and Physiotherapy
University of Nottingham

and

PAM McCLINTON

Head of Palliative Care and Clinical Quality/Nurse Advisor
Sue Ryder Care Central Office, London

Foreword by
ROGER BARKER

Cambridge Centre for Brain Repair
Department of Clinical Neuroscience, University of Cambridge
Addenbrooke's Hospital, Cambridge

Radcliffe Publishing
Oxford • New York

Radcliffe Publishing Ltd
18 Marcham Road
Abingdon
Oxon OX14 1AA
United Kingdom

www.radcliffe-oxford.com

Electronic catalogue and worldwide online ordering facility.

British Library Cataloguing in Publication Data

A catalogue record for this book is available from the British Library.

ISBN-13: 978 184619 293 7

The paper used for the text pages of this book is FSC certified. FSC (The Forest Stewardship Council) is an international network to promote responsible management of the world's forests.

Mixed Sources
Product group from well-managed forests and other controlled sources
www.fsc.org Cert no. SGS-COC-2482
© 1996 Forest Stewardship Council

Typeset by Pindar NZ, Auckland, New Zealand
Printed and bound by TJI Digital, Padstow, Cornwall, UK

Contents

Foreword

'Palliative care is an important public health issue. It is concerned with the suffering, the dignity, the care needs and the quality of life of people at the end of their lives. It is also concerned with the care and support of their families and friends. This is by and large a neglected topic in Europe, but one that is relevant to everyone.'

(World Health Organization)

The perception and expectations in treating patients with long-term neurological disorders is changing. It has moved from an area of diagnosis and therapeutic nihilism to one of holistic practice and for those involved in this area of medical practice there is an increasing need to a be a part of this transition. This book helps enormously in this respect.

Chronic long-term neurological disorders, especially those of neurodegenerative origin, tend to be managed by neurologists, old age psychiatrists and physicians involved with the care for the elderly, and in some cases by paediatric neurologists. Each of these disciplines has areas of expertise – the neurologists and psychiatrists in diagnosis and drug treatment; the care of the elderly physician with the management and social support of patients; and the paediatric neurologists with diagnosis and management including the family in those discussions. In addition, all of these disciplines refer, with little encouragement, to such relevant and helpful disciplines as physiotherapy, speech and language therapy and occupational therapy. However, as the disease progresses more input is required of a palliative nature. This may be within a respite or nursing home placement and the various specialists often feel this is not their responsibility, in part because they feel much less confident in this aspect of patient care. This is in contrast to other areas of medicine, most notably cancer, where palliative care is well established and factored early into the care package of patients. This point has been recently reinforced by Terry Pratchett, when writing about the future of his own case of Alzheimer's disease.

All of the major neurodegenerative disorders of the central nervous system (CNS), such as Alzheimer's and Parkinson's disease, are currently incurable and will lead to death. This can greatly reduce the life expectancy of some patients especially those where the condition presents earlier (e.g. Huntington's disease) or progresses rapidly (e.g. motor neurone disease). Thus all of those who interact with such patients will at some point have to engage with end of life issues, however difficult this may seem. Indeed in the modern age there is almost a belief that death should be curable and that a failure to deliver on such a therapy is a failing of the medical profession, rather than an inevitable failure of the complex biological systems of our bodies and brain.

This book confronts and deals with these topics of palliative care and end of life issues in long-term neurological disorders and does so in a wonderfully helpful way. This involves not only a helpful discussion about the issues and how to approach them, but it also gets us to admit and accept that the optimal management of such patients involves being part of a team, each member of which brings their own area of unique expertise. Nowhere is this more pertinent than the period concluding life.

We can see end of life management as an acknowledgement of our failure and thus portray it as a negative experience that conveys hopelessness as we sign off the individual to the inevitability of death. However, what we often forget is that end of life issues will be played out in us all, and that there are many experts who can bring huge help to those at this stage of life, including all those suffering from their chronic degenerative neurological conditions. It can therefore be a very positive and helpful experience that many find extremely beneficial, and which many of us are rather ignorant about.

I remember my own inadequacies in trying to deal with cases of advanced juvenile Huntington's disease – in particular the problems of managing symptoms and problems in a one young individual, only to have my eyes opened by a palliative care consultant, who had been involved in a similar case for several years. Such was my level of naivety that I thought that such specialists only got involved when patients were transferred to hospices for the very end of life – namely the last few weeks.

Living with neurological disease is not easy, especially when it involves mental as well as physical problems. However, recognising how it will evolve and what the issues are is important in best managing patients and the families in which they are embedded. To avoid the palliative aspects of medical practice and end of life issues is not an option for those who see patients with these disorders. The numbers of such cases will increase as the population ages and the development of specialist clinics in which to manage them is to be applauded, but dealing with the disorder from diagnosis to death is necessary and does not just involve different drugs.

This book provides a unique insight into the very real challenges of palliative care and end of life issues in patients with neurodegenerative disorders of the CNS, and I have found it a profoundly helpful read – not least in highlighting just how much I avoid these issues in my own practice, and how little I know about them.

Dr Roger Barker BA MBBS MRCP PhD
Cambridge Centre for Brain Repair
Department of Clinical Neuroscience, University of Cambridge
Addenbrooke's Hospital, Cambridge
June 2009

Preface

It is only in recent years that there has been serious attention paid to how a palliative care approach can be applied to people affected by conditions other than cancer, and to the specific challenges involved in palliative care delivery for distinct groups of patients. However, there is little empirical evidence identifying the palliative and end of life care needs of people and their families living with progressive long-term neurological conditions (PLTNCs) and how these can be addressed. Edited by a multidisciplinary team from Sue Ryder Care and the Sue Ryder Care Centre for Palliative and End of Life Studies at the University of Nottingham, and drawing on contributions from the experiences of doctors, nurses and the wider multidisciplinary team, this book aims to provide an accessible text for health and social care professionals caring for people with palliative and end of life care needs as a result of PLTNCs, focusing on the following four conditions: motor neurone disease (MND), multiple sclerosis (MS), Parkinson's disease (PD) and Huntington's disease (HD) and closely related disorders.

In their advanced stages people with PLTNCs present a range of problems which may make both care delivery and advance planning for care in the last stages of life both complex and challenging: ethically, practically and clinically. This is due to the range of physical, cognitive and emotional problems that people experience as they approach the end of their lives, as well as challenges relating to communication, decision making about nutrition and technologies of life support, and family care.

Contributors to this book recognise that people may require intensive input from rehabilitation and therapy teams at the same time as complex symptom management and supportive non clinical care. However, given that palliative care needs among people with PLTNCs may be present from diagnosis, it is the integration of palliative care and neurological expertise which is the focus of this book.

We recognise the complex issues of care coordination, communication and the need for team working when caring for people with PLTNCs and aim to provide an accessible and relevant overview of how a palliative care approach can enhance the experience of giving and receiving care for those affected by PLTNCs.

We hope that those reading this book will be inspired to seek out ways to address such complex issues and be encouraged to build bridges between palliative and neurological care to enable people with PLTNCs to live with the best quality of life for as long as possible.

Judi Byrne
Penny McNamara
Jane Seymour
Pam McClinton
June 2009

PALLIATIVE CARE IN NEUROLOGICAL DISEASE

Sue Ryder Care is a national charity providing compassionate health and social care to people across the UK.

We provide three types of health and social care: homecare, palliative and end of life, and neurological care. Our homecare supports people needing support and their families. Our palliative care ensures people receive compassionate, timely and expert support at all stages of illness and our neurological care provides services for complex late stage conditions when people can no longer be cared for at home.

For information about our work contact: 0845 050 1953 or email: info@suerydercare.org

About the editors

Judi Byrne has a wide level of experience and knowledge of operational management within the NHS, charity and commercial environment. Her work on developing palliative care pathways for cancer patients has led to a focus on the issues and challenges in providing care for everyone at the end of life, not just those with a cancer diagnosis. Currently she leads on the national PINC Care at the End of Life programme for Sue Ryder Care, which has been recognised in the NHS National End of Life Care Strategy as an example of good practice.

Penny McNamara is a consultant in palliative medicine at St John's Hospice Sue Ryder Care and Bedford NHS Trust. She spent much of her early medical training in the South Thames region, before moving to East Anglia when her husband took up his consultant post in anaesthesia at Bedford Hospital. She became interested in medical ethics at medical school and completed her thesis for her MSc around the issues of rationing as applied to palliative care. She contributed to the ethics chapter in the *Oxford Handbook of Palliative Care* and has published work on management of malignant ascites and fractured neck of femurs in patients with advanced malignancy.

She is currently the Programme Director for SpR training in Palliative Medicine in the Eastern Deanery and chairs the development group.

Jane Seymour is head of the Sue Ryder Care Centre in Palliative and End of Life Studies at the University of Nottingham. She has a nursing and social science background and has been a researcher and teacher in palliative and end of life care since 1994, following a career in clinical nursing. Jane's current research interests focus primarily on the development of palliative care beyond cancer care, advance care planning, older people's experiences of end of life care and public and professional education in these areas. She has published widely in the nursing, social science and palliative care press on these themes.

Pam McClinton qualified as a Registered Nurse and worked as a staff nurse and ward sister before moving to work in the community and complete further training to be a district nurse. It was while working as a district nurse that her interest in palliative care developed and she progressed to become a Community Macmillan Nurse. Her interest and expertise in palliative care continued as she chaired the Royal College of Nursing Palliative Nurses Forum and also worked as a Macmillan Lecturer at the Centre for Cancer and Palliative Care Studies based at the Royal Marsden Hospital. Recently she has been part of the National Audit Office expert panel on end of life care.

List of contributors

Ms Aimee Aubeeluck
Faculty of Medicine and Health Sciences
School of Nursing, Derbyshire Royal Infirmary
Derby

Dr Francesca Crawley
Consultant in Neurology
West Suffolk Hospital
Bury St Edmunds, West Suffolk

Mrs Lorraine Dixon
Palliative Care Services Manager
Leckhampton Court Hospice
Leckhampton, Gloucestershire

Ms Elaine Duro
Faculty of Medicine and Health Sciences
School of Nursing, Derbyshire Royal Infirmary
Derby

Dr Annette Edwards
Consultant in Palliative Medicine
Sue Ryder Care
Wheatfields Hospice, Leeds

Mr Craig Maddock
Staff Nurse
Leckhampton Court Hospice
Leckhampton, Gloucestershire

Dr Richard Partridge
Macmillan/Sue Ryder Care Consultant in Palliative Medicine
Sue Ryder Care
Thorpe Hall Hospice, Peterborough, Cambridgeshire

Ms Kim Wilcox
Staff Nurse, Leckhampton Court Hospice
Leckhampton, Gloucestershire

Ms Eleanor Wilson
Research Fellow/PhD student
Sue Ryder Care Centre for Palliative and End of Life Studies
School of Nursing, Queen's Medical Centre, Nottingham

CHAPTER 1

Progressive neurological conditions: epidemiological and clinical picture

Francesca Crawley

There are many different progressive long-term neurological conditions (PLTNCs). This chapter focuses on multiple sclerosis (MS) and Parkinson's disease (PD), which are two of the more common conditions, and on motor neurone disease (MND) and Huntington's disease (HD), which are much rarer. In the UK, each general practitioner will have an average of three people with MS on their case load, but only a one in ten chance of a patient with MND.

Reference is made in this chapter to the 'incidence' and the 'prevalence' of each disease. The 'incidence' is the number of new cases of the disease developing in a year and the 'prevalence' is the number of patients with that disease at any point in time.

MULTIPLE SCLEROSIS
Epidemiology of MS

Multiple sclerosis (MS) is the most common central nervous system disease to affect young adults. It is more common in women than in men (2:1). Disease onset is generally in the third or fourth decade of life.

There is no database of patients with MS in the UK. We base our estimate of the total number of individuals with the disease on local population studies, extrapolated to include the whole country. By using these estimates, there are thought to be about 85 000 people with MS in the UK. Worldwide the prevalence is thought to be around 2 500 000. In the UK we think that about 2500 people are diagnosed with MS each year.[1]

People with MS are not distributed evenly throughout the world. The prevalence of the disease increases as you travel further away (north or south) from the equator. For example, in the UK, this means that there are more people with

MS per 1000 of the population in northern Scotland than in London. Looking more globally, the incidence is higher in Canada than in an equatorial country such as India.

The risk of developing MS if you move from a low risk part of the world, for example India, to a high risk part of the world, for example the UK, depends on the age at which you migrate. If you move as a child, your risk will become similar to that of others living in the country to which you move, but if you move as an adult you maintain the level of risk from your native country. This shows the interaction of genetic and environmental factors on the risk of developing this disease.

In general in the UK, the risk of developing MS is about one in 700. In addition to this risk varying with where in the UK an individual lives, it is also increased by having family members with the disease. If you have a first degree relative (parent, sibling, child) with MS, your risk of developing the disease is one in 40, and if you have a second degree relative (cousins, aunts/uncles, nephews/nieces) it is one in 100.[2] MS is a progressive neurological disorder which people often live with for many years. Overall, an individual's life expectancy is only slightly shortened by MS, although this varies greatly from one individual to another.

The precise environmental factors which trigger MS remain largely unknown and multiple studies have had conflicting results. Possible triggers which have been identified include age at infection by Epstein Barr virus and climate induced changes in vitamin D levels. None of the theories are proven.

Pathology of MS

It is thought that MS is caused by the body's own cells attacking cells within the central nervous system (CNS). This is called an autoimmune reaction. The attacking cells are a type of white blood cell called T lymphocytes. These T lymphocytes enter the CNS and attack the myelin which surrounds the cell. This is called demyelination. When myelin is damaged the nerve impulse cannot pass so easily down the nerve cell. This means that messages cannot get through to the correct place. For example, if there is damaged myelin between the pathway from the brain to the legs, walking is likely to be difficult. If the myelin is damaged between the brain and the eye, vision will be affected.

In the early stages of MS, remyelination can occur. This means that the damaged myelin can be repaired. However, the repaired myelin is often thinner and does not conduct the nerve impulses as well as the original myelin did. Over time however, the cells that produce myelin (oligodendrocytes) become damaged and myelin is not replaced. The nerve which was protected by the myelin (the axon), then dies. If just a small part of the axon dies, the CNS is able to reroute messages, however, if it is a larger area of damage the rerouting can not happen and the pathway is permanently blocked.

Types of MS

Most people with MS have relapsing remitting MS at the onset of their disease. This means that they develop a neurological problem which persists for a while (usually a few weeks; the relapse) and then recover (the remission). It is easy to understand what is happening pathologically.

In the relapse, there is demyelination. Once remyelination has occurred there is a remission from the symptoms. For the purpose of clinical trials, a relapse has been defined as lasting more than 24 hours in the context of a normal body temperature and that to consider attacks to be separate they should be at least 30 days apart.[3]

The severity, the frequency and the gap between relapses is hugely variable and impossible to predict. Most people with relapsing remitting MS have one or two relapses a year. Over years, this pattern of disease may change into progressive MS. Here relapses become less frequent, but disability increases. This is termed 'secondary progressive MS'.

Studies suggest that people who initially have relapsing remitting MS develop secondary progressive MS after about 10 years.[4] Other individuals develop progressive MS from disease onset. This is called primary progressive MS. These individuals tend to be older at the time of disease onset, with a mean age of onset about 40 years. A final type of MS is benign MS. Here attacks are mild and often years apart.

Symptoms from MS

Symptoms in MS depend on the part of the nervous system in which demyelination occurs. For example, the optic nerve, which relays visual information from the eye to the brain, is often affected. This is usually only one eye and causes a painful reduction in vision. Colour vision is often particularly affected. Alternatively, demyelination in the balance area of the brain (the cerebellum), causes difficulty walking, slurred speech and problems with coordination. Involvement of the part of the brain that is involved in sensation causes numbness or tingling. If the patient is not seen acutely, these signs have often resolved by the time they are seen in clinic.

Other symptoms from MS include bowel and bladder disturbance, memory problems, depression and personality change. Fatigue is also common, affecting up to 75% of patients.[5] Many patients rate fatigue as their main problem in MS. This type of fatigue differs from the fatigue experienced in depression. MS associated fatigue is often worse with heat, exercise or later in the day and is often relieved by a short rest. Depression associated fatigue is more non specific and often associated with other depressive symptoms such as sleep disturbance. Many of these symptoms come and go in the initial phases of the disease, but as MS progresses, symptoms and therefore disability, accrue.

Diagnosis of MS

Patients with primary progressive MS usually present with a gait disorder. This has often come on very gradually and the individual has adapted to maintain functional ability. These individuals often have very abnormal neurological examinations at their first presentation in an outpatient clinic.

MS is often suspected by a clinician on the basis of the history and examination of the patient, but investigations are mandatory. Magnetic resonance imaging (MRI) is now the most standard investigation. Imaging of the brain and sometimes the spinal cord is performed. Typically, MS causes lesions in the white matter of the brain, particularly around the ventricles. Gadolinium enhancement is seen with lesions which are less than about 4–6 weeks old. These new enhancing lesions are about 5–10 times more common than the clinical relapse frequency. For this reason, they have been used as surrogate markers in clinical trials. In the right clinical context these can be diagnostic, but if there is any doubt a lumbar puncture is performed to examine the cerebrospinal fluid for the presence of oligoclonal bands. These can be found in other neurological diseases other than MS but up to 95% of patients with clinically definite MS will have them.[6]

Electrical tests (evoked responses) are occasionally done. These involve examining the conduction time in a nerve or nerves. Demyelination causes slowing of the impulse and thus a prolonged conduction time. Blood tests are required to exclude other conditions which may mimic MS.

Initial treatment of MS

The initial management of MS involves explaining the diagnosis to the patient. It is desirable that this is done by a member of the neurological team who has enough experience to be able to answer any questions accurately. Many patients find early involvement with an MS nurse to be of great benefit. Some MS centres run courses over a series of evenings to introduce patients and relatives to the nature of MS and to educate them about different aspects of the disease.

Initially, relapses are often treated with steroids. These are increasingly given as oral tablets (methylprednisolone). Methylprednisolone speeds up recovery from an individual relapse, but does not alter the final outcome. There is no effect on long-term disability. Various studies have shown a role for disease modifying drugs in the management of MS. These include interferon,[7,8,9] CAMPATH, natalizumab[10] and mitoxantrone.[11] These drugs are used in an attempt to prevent disease progression: both relapse rate and disability. In the UK, they are available via specialist MS clinics; sometimes via clinical trials. The ideal treatment would stop relapses, halt disease progression and reverse any disability: unfortunately we do not yet have such a drug.

Symptomatic treatment is also commonly employed in MS. For example, pain may be managed with conventional painkillers such as paracetamol or anti inflammatory drugs, or with less conventional drugs, such as anticonvulsants and antidepressants. Bladder involvement is often best managed by a continence advisor, often in the community. This may involve drugs or sometimes catheterisation. For some individuals self catheterisation can be done a couple of times a day, thus draining the bladder effectively but avoiding a permanent catheter.

Depression is often treated with antidepressant tablets and with psychological support, if this is available locally. Fatigue can sometimes be helped with medication, but is often best managed by a more pragmatic approach. In such an approach, education of all parties (patient, carer, and employer) to maximise flexibility and to pace day to day activities can be beneficial. For example, an afternoon sleep may help tremendously, but some patients need encouragement to take this. Similarly, an employer may agree to this if the importance and benefit is explained.

At many stages of MS, the involvement of the specialist therapist, including physiotherapists, occupational therapists and speech and language therapists is tremendously important. For example, a physiotherapist may be able to preserve independent walking and at another stage in the disease may offer advice on a wheelchair. Occupational therapists may look at adapting an individual's home, to enable him or her to live there more safely. Speech and language therapists are often involved in assessing swallowing.

MOTOR NEURONE DISEASE
Epidemiology of MND

In contrast to MS, motor neurone disease (MND) is a rare disease. The incidence is 1.5–2 in 100 000 and the prevalence 5–7 in 100 000. There are two men affected for every woman.[12] It tends to affect older people, with a peak age at diagnosis of 55–75 years. It does, however, occasionally occur in people in their 20s. Stephen Hawking, the world famous physicist is such an example.

The incidence of MND is 50–150 times higher in the Western Pacific than in the rest of the world. This is possibly due to toxins in seeds such as the cycad. Five per cent of the disease is genetic in origin. The only mutation identified to date is the superoxide dismutase gene, which is autosomal dominant. Autosomal dominant means that if an individual has the gene he or she will develop the disease and it will be passed down to a quarter of any children that they may have.

MND generally shortens life expectancy; with the average length of remaining life being two years from diagnosis, but this is hugely variable.

Pathology of MND

In MND, motor neurones degenerate. These can be in the brain cortex, brainstem, spinal cord and corticospinal tract. It is not known what causes this degeneration. There is no repair process and so, in contrast to MS, the disease is generally progressive from onset. The parts of the nervous system which are involved in bowel and bladder function, the sensory system and control of eye movements are not affected by MND.

Types of MND

The most common type of MND is amyotrophic lateral sclerosis (ALS). In this form of MND there is involvement of both upper and lower motor neurones. Upper motor neurones are those nerve cells from the brain to the spinal cord and lower motor neurones are those from the spinal cord to the muscles. Therefore, in ALS, there is a mixture of upper and lower motor problems.

Alternatively, there may just be upper motor neurone involvement. This is termed 'primary lateral sclerosis'. Pure lower motor neurone disease also occurs, generally presenting with difficulties speaking or swallowing.

Symptoms from MND

People with MND present with a variety of different symptoms. Weakness and difficulty walking are common. This often only involves one leg at disease onset. Another common symptom is difficulty using a hand, for example to do fiddly tasks such as buttons. Speech may be affected and the patient notices slurred speech or may describe difficulty with articulation. Swallowing problems such as choking may be the first symptom. As the disease progresses, new symptoms develop. This may be rapid, for example over weeks. Alternatively, disease progression can be slower, over months. Vision, sensation and continence are not affected by MND. Cognition and memory can be affected, but this is often difficult to disentangle from any speech disturbance.

Respiratory function is commonly affected. Individuals become aware of opthopnoea (difficulty breathing when lying flat). Often, breathing at night is affected and this can lead to a raised level of carbon dioxide in the blood stream. This may then lead to poor nocturnal sleep and therefore daytime sleepiness or headache.

Diagnosis of MND

MND is a fatal condition and accurate diagnosis is essential. The El Escorial criteria[13] for diagnosis of MND are widely accepted as the gold standard for diagnosis. However, these were designed for research and clinical trials and often are not fulfilled in clinical practice.

Practically, diagnosis includes nerve conduction studies and electromyogram, looking for evidence of MND and imaging, blood tests and possibly a lumbar puncture, to look for evidence of any other disease. Diagnostic difficulty is common, particularly in people with only upper or lower motor neurone signs, rather than a mixture.

Explaining a diagnosis of MND requires a neurologist with experience of this condition. There needs to be a provisional plan agreed with the patient; whether it is referral to specialist therapists, involvement of an MND care coordinator, referral to a respiratory team or all of these. Follow up generally needs to be fairly rapid, either by the neurologist or another experienced member of the MND team. Many areas now have specialist MND clinics, run by one or two neurologists from the centre in conjunction with a speech and language therapist, dietician, physiotherapist, palliative care doctor or nurse, among others. This multidisciplinary team can generally offer patients with MND the best hope of maintaining quality of life in the face of rapidly changing disability.

Initial treatment of MND

Riluzole is the only drug licensed to treat MND. Riluzole inhibits the release of glutamate and neuronal damage in vitro. It is disease modifying, rather than symptomatic. Riluzole has been shown to prolong survival in individuals who present without bulbar (speech and swallowing) involvement by a few months.[14,15] It is generally well tolerated. Many neurologists prescribe the drug as a means of offering the patient hope, rather than any physical benefit.

Recent studies have demonstrated that non invasive ventilation can both prolong survival and, probably more importantly, improve quality of life of both carer and patient in certain individuals with MND.[16,17] Ventilatory capacity is usually assessed via specialised breathing tests, often in specialist clinics. The non invasive ventilators are portable and require use of a face mask. Many individuals initially use non invasive ventilation either just at night, or only when feeling short of breath, although others come to rely on the machine for 24 hours a day.

Nutrition is another issue in MND. Swallowing can be affected at any stage of the disease. Specialist speech and language therapists provide swallow assessments and guide management. Initially, a modified diet, for example with soft food, may be appropriate, but eventually supplementary enteral feeding is often needed. This is usually provided via a tube inserted via the abdomen into the stomach, bypassing the need to swallow. There are two methods of inserting such a tube; either endoscopically or radiologically. The tube can be used to 'top up' calories, or to provide all nutrition and fluids. Specialist MND services generally aim to discuss placement of these tubes while the patient is relatively well, rather than later in the disease when the position is more precarious.

People with MND, like MS, often require a multidisciplinary team of therapists. However, because of the very poor prognosis and often rapidly changing disability, these therapists are often very closely involved with each patient from diagnosis to death.

PARKINSON'S DISEASE

Parkinson's disease (PD) was originally described by James Parkinson in an essay describing the triad of tremor, rigidity and bradykinesia.[18]

Epidemiology

The incidence of PD is about 300 per 100 000 population. The incidence increases with age. It generally presents above the age of 50 years. Two thirds of patients are over 70 years old. The lifetime risk of developing PD is estimated to be 2% for men and 1.3% for women.[18] Several studies have suggested that Caucasians are affected more than African Americans, but this is not confirmed. The lack of uniform diagnostic criteria may partially explain a variable incidence rate in different cultures.

Various studies have examined both the risk of smoking and consumption of alcohol on subsequent development of PD. This data suggests that smoking may be protective.[19] Population studies have demonstrated that PD is more common in industrial societies than in rural ones,[20] and is more common in North America and Europe than in the Far East.

PD is sometimes inherited. The first gene which causes PD was identified in 1997[21] and several more have been discovered since. Some of these are dominant and others recessively inherited.

Pathology of PD

PD is marked by the degeneration of dopamine containing cells in the pars compacta of the substantia nigra. Cell loss also occurs in other pigmented brain stem nuclei, autonomic nuclei and pyramidal cells.

Presentation of PD

PD classically presents with the triad of tremor, rigidity and bradykinesia, as described originally by James Parkinson. At disease onset, these symptoms are generally unilateral. Retrospectively, the individual may have noticed various symptoms for several years pre diagnosis, including stiffness, joint pain, difficulty with writing and increasing immobility. These are often misdiagnosed as 'arthritis' or 'ageing'. The presence of rest tremor (i.e. tremor which is present when the patient is relaxed, rather than when attempting to do a motor task) often alerts the clinician to the correct diagnosis. Posture is often stooped and walking slow and shuffling. Speech may become monotonous and quiet. Facial expression and eye movements are reduced. These signs may initially be subtle.

Later in PD the signs are more evident. Walking becomes very slow and freezing may develop. This describes interruption of the normal gait and inability to continue. Balance may worsen and falls develop. Swallowing can be problematic. Cognitive disturbance is often initially manifested as hallucinations. These are generally visual and non threatening. Later on, a dementia may occur.

Sleep disturbance is common in PD. Individuals develop a REM (rapid eye movement) sleep disturbance, with vivid dreams, shouting and even lashing out at a partner during sleep. This is often not volunteered by patients, unless specifically asked about.

Other common problems associated with PD include constipation, greasy skin, depression, mood disturbance (particularly depression), sexual dysfunction, urological disturbance, swallowing difficulties and autonomic disturbance.

Diagnosis of PD

PD is generally a clinical diagnosis. The differential diagnosis may include essential tremor, drug induced parkinsonism and vascular parkinsonism.

Occasionally ioflupane is used diagnostically. This is a nuclear medical neuro imaging technique, looking at dopaminergic reuptake within the brain.

Initial management of PD

In the UK, the initial management of PD generally focuses on explanation and details of support and information such as can be obtained via the Parkinson's Disease Society. Drugs are often not needed initially. As symptoms progress and everyday life is affected, the need for drug therapy is reviewed. Levodopa is the mainstay of drug therapy. This is given in combination with a drug to enable levodopa to pass through the gut without being metabolised. After a period of some years, patients often develop problems with levodopa, including rapid peak and trough drug concentrations which result in periods of excess mobility (dyskinesias) and the immobility (freezing). An alternative and sometimes additional drug strategy uses dopamine agonists. There is some evidence that if these drugs are used initially, the long-term problems with levodopa can at least be delayed. However, they are often not powerful enough drugs to control disease symptomatology. Generally, dopamine agonists are used first line in patients who are younger at disease onset. Other drugs may include amantadine for mild bradykinesia and rigidity and anticholinergics for young patients with tremor.

Neurosurgical techniques are emerging as treatment for PD. These are generally reserved for individuals with advanced disease. In the UK there are stringent guidelines from the National Institute for Health and Clinical Excellence (NICE) regarding these treatments.

HUNTINGTON'S DISEASE

Huntington's disease (HD) is an autosomal dominant condition. It causes a movement disorder and cognitive changes. It is progressive and causes premature death.

Epidemiology of HD

HD is a genetically determined, autosomal dominant condition. This means that half of the offspring of affected individuals are likely to develop the condition. It can occur sporadically, but if an accurate history is taken, there is often premature death of a parent or non paternity in these cases. The prevalence in the UK is 4–10 per 100 000.[22]

It is known that HD is caused by an unstable trinucleotide repeat on chromosome 4.[23] All individuals with the disease have more than 35 repeats. The number of repeats in an individual reflects the age at presentation of the disease. HD shows anticipation, meaning that it can present at an earlier age in successive generations. The trinucleotide repeat encodes a protein called Huntingtin.

Pathology of HD

This can be very variable. In the most advanced cases there is atrophy of parts of the basal ganglia (caudate and putamen) and of the cortex and subcortical structures. However, some asymptomatic individuals can have widespread pathological changes, while other symptomatic ones have little in the way of abnormal findings.

Presentation of HD

Unfortunately, HD often presents in an individual with a family history of the disease who is well aware what the diagnosis is likely to be. The disease onset can be at any age from childhood to old age. Most patients are 30–50 years at onset.[22]

Two thirds of patients initially notice motor problems, mainly chorea. This is an involuntary writhing movement of the limbs and/or trunk. There may be additional bradykinesia (slowness of movements) and rigidity.[24] The disease progresses to result in increasing immobility, falls and speech and swallowing difficulties. Weight loss can be problematic, both due to the chorea itself and to the difficulty in swallowing.

In the other third of individuals the initial symptoms are cognitive. Initially, there is irritability, apathy, anxiety and altered mood. Work may be affected, finances may suffer and family relationships deteriorate. Depression is common and may lead to self harm. Dementia may become apparent.

Diagnosis of HD

HD is generally a genetic diagnosis. This means analysis of the patient's DNA. Generally this is only performed following genetic counselling either by a geneticist or by a neurologist with a particular interest in HD. As in all genetic diagnoses, there are widespread implications for the family. In patients under 50 years it is always important to exclude Wilson's disease. This can also present with a movement disorder and cognitive changes. It is a disorder of copper metabolism and is fairly straightforward to diagnose via biochemical tests.

Initial management of HD

There is no disease modifying treatment for HD. The movement disorder can be helped by tetrabenazine or neuroleptic drugs. Depression should be treated appropriately. Psychosis may require neuroleptics. From the initial diagnosis a multidisciplinary team approach is required, usually involving a neurologist, physiotherapist, occupational therapist, speech and language therapist and dietician. These are often under the umbrella of a specialist HD clinic. Psychiatric and palliative care involvement is often required early in the disease, involving a combination of community, respite and long-term care provision.

CONCLUSION

PLTNCs are very varied in their presentation, rate of progression and effect on lifespan. In this chapter we have concentrated on and outlined the epidemiology, pathology and route to diagnosis of multiple sclerosis, Parkinson's disease, motor neurone disease, and Huntington's disease. These diseases have many differences from each other, but also share similar problems and cause common challenges to those affected. Similar to other PLTNCs, and as patients reach the palliative phases of these diseases, they all require a multidisciplinary approach in order to reduce their disability and suffering.

REFERENCES

1 Compston A, Confavreux C. The distribution of multiple sclerosis. In: *McAlpine's Multiple Sclerosis*. 4th ed. London: Churchill Livingstone; 2005. pp. 71–111.

2 Compston A, Wekerle, H. The genetics of multiple sclerosis. In: *McAlpine's Multiple Sclerosis*. 4th ed. London: Churchill Livingstone; 2005. pp. 113–81.

3 Palace J. Making the diagnosis of multiple sclerosis. *J Neurol Neurosurg Psychiatry.* 2001; 71(Suppl. 2): ii, 3–8.

4 Lublin FD, Reingold SC. Defining the clinical course of multiple sclerosis: results of an international survey. National Multiple Sclerosis Society (USA) Advisory Committee on Clinical Trials of New Agents in Multiple Sclerosis. *Neurol.* 1996; 46(4): 907–11.

5 Edgley K, Sullivan M, Dehoux E. A survey of multiple sclerosis: determination of employment status. *Can J Rehab.* 1991; 4: 127–32.

6 McLean BN, Luxton RW, Thompson EJ. A study of immunoglobulin G in the cerebrospinal fluid of 1007 patients with suspected neurological disease using isoelectric focusing and the Log IgG-Index: a comparison and diagnostic applications. *Brain.* 1990; 113(Pt 5): 1269–89.

7 Jacobs LD, Cookfair DL, Rudick RA, *et al.* Intramuscular interferon beta-1a for disease progression in relapsing multiple sclerosis. The Multiple Sclerosis Collaborative Research Group (MSCRG). *Ann Neurol.* 1996; 39(3): 285–94.

8 PRISMS (Prevention of Relapses and Disability by Interferon beta-1a Subcutaneously in Multiple Sclerosis) Study Group. Randomised double-blind placebo-controlled study of interferon beta-1a in relapsing/remitting multiple sclerosis. *Lancet.* 1998; 352(9139): 1498–504.

9 IFNB Multiple Sclerosis Study Group. Interferon beta-1b is effective in relapsing-remitting multiple sclerosis. I. Clinical results of a multicenter, randomized, double-blind, placebo-controlled trial. *Neurol.* 1993; 43(4): 655–61.

10 Miller DH, Khan OA, Sheremata WA, *et al.* A controlled trial of natalizumab for relapsing multiple sclerosis. *N Engl J Med.* 2003; 348(1): 15–23.

11 Hartung HP, Gonsette R, Konig N, *et al.* Mitoxantrone in progressive multiple sclerosis: a placebo-controlled, double-blind, randomised, multicentre trial. *Lancet.* 2002; 360(9350): 2018–25.

12 Kahana E, Alter M, Feldman S. Amyotrophic lateral sclerosis: a population study. *J Neurol.* 1976; 212(3): 205–13.

13 Brooks BR, Miller RG, Swash M, *et al.* El Escorial revisited: revised criteria for the diagnosis of amyotrophic lateral sclerosis. *Amyotroph Lateral Scler Other Motor Neuron Disord.* 2000; 1(5): 293–9.

14 Lacomblez L, Bensimon G, Leigh PN, *et al.* Dose-ranging study of riluzole in amyotrophic lateral sclerosis. Amyotrophic Lateral Sclerosis/Riluzole Study Group II. *Lancet.* 1996; 347(9013): 1425–31.

15 Bensimon G, Lacomblez L, Meininger V. A controlled trial of riluzole in amyotrophic lateral sclerosis. ALS/Riluzole Study Group. *N Engl J Med.* 1994; 330(9): 585–91.

16 Servera E, Sancho J. Non-invasive ventilation in amyotrophic lateral sclerosis. *Lancet Neurol.* 2006; 5(4): 291–2; author reply 292–3.

17 Bourke SC, Tomlinson M, Williams TL, *et al.* Effects of non-invasive ventilation on survival and quality of life in patients with amyotrophic lateral sclerosis: a randomised controlled trial. *Lancet Neurol.* 2006; 5(2): 140–7.

18 Elbaz A, Bower JH, Maraganore DM, *et al.* Risk tables for parkinsonism and Parkinson's disease. *J Clin Epidemiol.* 2002; 55(1): 25–31.

19 Elbaz A, Manubens-Bertran JM, Baldereschi M, *et al.* Parkinson's disease, smoking, and family history. EUROPARKINSON Study Group. *J Neurol.* 2000; 247(10): 793–8.

20 Rajput AH. Environmental causation of Parkinson's disease. *Arch Neurol.* 1993; 50(6): 651–2.

21 Polymeropoulos MH, Lavedan C, Leroy E, *et al.* Mutation in the alpha-synuclein gene identified in families with Parkinson's disease. *Science.* 1997; 276(5321): 2045–7.

22 Harper PS. The natural history of Huntington's disease. In: Harper PS. *Huntington's Disease.* London: WB Saunders; 1991. pp. 127–40.

23 Huntington's Disease Collaborative Research Group. A novel gene containing a trinucleotide repeat that is expanded and unstable on Huntington's disease chromosomes. *Cell.* 1993; 72(6): 971–83.

24 Thompson PD, Beradelli A, Rothwell JC, *et al.* The coexistence of bradykinesia and chorea in Huntington's disease and its implications for theories of basal ganglia control of movement. *Brain.* 1988; 111: 223–44.

CHAPTER 2

The principles and practice of palliative care

Jane Seymour

The principles of what we now call 'palliative care' have fascinating historical roots extending far back into ancient times when the very foundations of medicine and the caring professions were laid. These principles were reformulated in the mid 20th century to inform a distinct field of clinical practice, initially known as 'hospice' or 'terminal' care, which, to begin with, was predominantly focused on the needs of people affected by cancer. This field of practice rapidly diversified and expanded in the latter years of the 20th century across many different countries of the world. As we approach the end of the first decade of the 21st century, the provision of palliative care is beginning to feature in the political and policy agendas of many different countries as they seek to respond to the challenges of epidemiological and socio demographic change. The changing age structure of the countries in the developed world has given rise to a growth of palliative care needs among older people, often in association with diseases other than cancer; while younger people with complex palliative care needs due to life limiting disease or disability are living longer than at any time previously due to changes in medical technology. In the resource poor nations, the tragedies of the AIDS pandemic pose a challenge of gargantuan proportions, especially in Sub Saharan Africa.[1]

This chapter provides a brief overview of the history and recent development of palliative care internationally; summarises for readers some of the key dimensions of palliative care practice and philosophy; and sets out some important challenges for the provision of palliative care as it begins to expand beyond cancer care.

THE DEVELOPMENT OF PALLIATIVE CARE: A BRIEF HISTORICAL SKETCH

Clark and Seymour[2] have described how, during the 19th century and in the context of rising industrialisation and urbanisation in Europe and the beginnings of a growth of hospital medicine directed at curing and containing disease, there emerged a new social movement directed at the needs of the chronically sick, the aged, the dying and the poor. These groups of people were somewhat neglected in the newly emergent voluntary hospitals and, as a consequence of the gradual disappearance of traditional models of community and family based care for the dying, found themselves in dire need of support. Homes for the dying, sometimes called 'hospices', began to be established in Europe during the 19th and early 20th centuries, combining a focus on the care of people dying from tuberculosis and later cancer, with attention to relieving poverty. Among the most famous is St Joseph's Hospice in London, which celebrated its centenary in 2005.[3] In most cases, these institutions were founded by religious orders of women, such as the Sisters of Charity, who developed clinical practices in nursing which were to later have a major influence on the founder of the modern hospice movement, Cicely Saunders, and the related development of palliative care. Saunders, who was triply qualified as a nurse, medical social worker and doctor, founded St Christopher's Hospice, in Sydenham, London in 1967 to fulfil her vocation of applying all she had learnt in her varied career to relieve the suffering of patients with pain caused by cancer. This was the first 'modern hospice' in the world, thus called because it combined a philosophy of person centred care with the most advanced clinical techniques to control complex symptoms.[4] In the 1960s and 1970s, Saunders developed the notion of 'total pain' to capture an approach to care which is the essence of what was later called 'palliative care'. In this, the focus is towards the person and their experience of illness: emotionally, spiritually, and socially; rather than just the body and its manifestations of disease.[5]

Until the pioneering work of Saunders and like minded colleagues, there had been little medical interest in the treatment of the dying since the beginnings of a move towards hospital based medicine. Moreover, there were significant worries and concerns among all doctors practising in the mid 20th century about the use of opiates to relieve pain during dying; therefore many patients received little or no effective pain relief.[6] However, the work of Saunders and others drew inspiration from a residual clinical literature from the late 19th and early 20th centuries which was largely ignored by others in the race to adopt post Second World War 'scientific medicine'. This literature, which Saunders and others sought out, promoted a set of ideas about the value and necessity of clinicians accompanying and supporting dying patients, while also relieving pain and suffering using their clinical skills and resources in a pragmatic and adaptable manner.[6] A book written in the 1930s by an American physician, Alfred

Worcester, *The Care of the Aged, the Dying and the Dead*,[7] provides an insight into the key elements of their approach, with the most telling message being the idea that it 'matters much that we give ourselves with our pills'.[7]

The work of physicians such as Worcester was based on an Asklepian tradition of medicine stemming from Ancient Greece, in which the role of the clinician is to act as a healer, and to seek to empathically understand the suffering and experience of illness for the person for whom they cared, and to create a safe and secure environment for them.[8] This strand has been an important feature of palliative care philosophy since its inception, but Saunders and her colleagues never lost sight of what could also be contributed to excellent patient care by advances in medical science.[2,6] But possibly their greatest achievement was to have a broad scope of vision beyond medicine. As palliative care took shape as a distinct field of practice it developed a multidisciplinary perspective which enabled it to benefit from the distinct skills and knowledge of colleagues in nursing and the other professions allied to medicine, and promulgated the benefits to be gained from working together for the benefit of those in need, as opposed to encouraging professional isolation and separation.[2,6]

Since the establishment of St Christopher's Hospice in London in 1967, hospice and palliative care has expanded worldwide in a variety of forms and become associated with an ever widening range of terms, some of which are the focus of fierce debate and discussion.[9] The next sections of this chapter turn to examine the diversification of hospice and palliative care and to set out what might be seen as a the key characteristics or dimensions of palliative care, wherever it is provided.

THE INTERNATIONAL SPREAD OF PALLIATIVE CARE

Clark has described, through an analysis of Cicely Saunders' correspondence, how she was not an isolated figure in her concerns to develop a new approach to the care of the dying, but rather part of a much wider social and clinical movement which extended internationally.[10] The principles that were initially developed at St Christopher's Hospice were gradually (although not always without a struggle or evenly) adopted in other hospices and in hospitals and community services both in Britain and elsewhere. By the mid 1990s there were palliative care services, either attached to hospices or operating from within community or hospital services, in every part of Britain. In addition, most other European countries had developed services. By the 2000s resource poor countries were also beginning to develop a network of services: some of these built on established islands of provision which had existed for many years (for example, in Poland and in parts of Africa), while others were completely new, emerging as one aspect of attempts to deal with the crisis of AIDS. Clark and Wright[11] have categorised hospice-palliative care development, country by country, throughout the world, depicting this development in a series of world and regional maps. They describe palliative care service development by means of a four stage typology: 1) no identified hospice-palliative care activity, 2) capacity building activity, but no service, 3) localised palliative care provision and 4) countries where palliative care activities are approaching integration with mainstream service providers.[11]

KEY DIMENSIONS OF CONTEMPORARY PALLIATIVE CARE

Palliative care is an important public health issue. It is concerned with the suffering, the dignity, the care needs and the quality of life of people at the end of their lives. It is also concerned with the care and support of their families and friends. This is by and large a neglected topic in Europe, but one that is relevant to everyone.[12]

The World Health Organization (WHO)[13] describes palliative care as an approach that improves the quality of life of individuals and their families facing the problems associated with life threatening illness through the prevention and relief of suffering by means of early identification and impeccable assessment and treatment of pain and other problems, physical, psychosocial and spiritual. Palliative care:

➤ provides relief from pain and other distressing symptoms
➤ affirms life and regards dying as a normal process
➤ intends neither to hasten nor postpone death
➤ integrates the psychological and spiritual aspects of patient care
➤ offers a support system to help patients live as actively as possible until death
➤ offers a support system to help the family cope during the patient's illness and in their own bereavement
➤ uses a team approach to address the needs of patients and their families, including bereavement counselling, if indicated
➤ will enhance quality of life, and may also positively influence the course of illness
➤ is applicable early in the course of illness, in conjunction with other therapies that are intended to prolong life, such as chemotherapy or radiation therapy, and includes those investigations needed to better understand and manage distressing clinical complications.[14]

The professionals involved in providing palliative care fall into two categories.
➤ Those providing general care to patients and their family carers, for example the GP or district nurse. General palliative care consists of a core set of knowledge and skills to be used by all health and social care staff involved in the care and support of those facing the end of life and their companions.

➤ Those who specialise in palliative care (consultants in palliative medicine, or clinical nurse specialists in palliative care – in the UK, some of these may be called Macmillan nurses). Specialist palliative care can be delivered in hospices, hospitals, at home or in care homes, and is often provided as a consultancy or advice service.

Referral to specialist palliative care services may be indicated if:
➤ one or more distressing symptoms prove difficult to control
➤ there is severe emotional distress associated with the patient's deterioration
➤ the patient's family or informal carers, particularly potentially vulnerable ones such as dependent children and/or elderly relatives, are experiencing severe distress.[14]

From the comprehensive definition of palliative care provided by the WHO it is possible to identify the major components which make up a palliative care philosophy of care, whether this is within a specialist service or as part of a modality of care in a non specialist palliative care service. Those services that are perhaps most distinctive in palliative care are the emphases on: the relief of suffering; the impeccable assessment and treatment of pain and other problems; the enhancement of quality of life; and team working. The chapter turns now to look at each of these in turn.

Suffering

In his study of suffering, the physician Eric Cassell[15] argues that suffering is experienced by persons, occurs when an impending destruction of the person is perceived and continues until the integrity of the person can be restored in some manner. Suffering, like pain, is what the person says it is: it cannot be determined by an outsider looking in, and it will not relate in any neat linear form to the intensity of pain, to the nature of disease or to the symptoms and problems that the person appears to have. Fear of the unknown, fear of pain, or issues of a deep seated biographical nature may be a powerful feature in suffering, together with loss of meaning, status or future that those who become seriously ill may have to endure. Illness means different things to different people,[16] and it is these meanings that relate to the experience of suffering and within which the keys to its relief are found. Helping the person who is suffering involves understanding what is a highly personal reaction to illness and distress. For some people, the experience of suffering is linked to a search for spiritual or religious explanations for questions that emerge from the experience of suffering: Why me? Why now? Why like this? For others, meaning will be sought in other terms – perhaps through relationships or particular activities that are important.

Assessment and treatment of pain

Although Saunders' use of the term 'Total Pain' has been criticised[17] as perhaps misrepresenting the multidimensional experience of suffering among seriously ill people, she probably used the term to bring to clinicians' attention, by using a language they understood, the need to consider physical pain as only one aspect of patients' experiences of distress. However, the relief of physical pain has always been considered as an essential first step in addressing the wider aspects of suffering. For reasons of space, the chapter therefore focuses on this issue. Readers should be aware that other chapters in this book address a wide range of other problems.

Until the 1960s, pain was considered by most clinicians as an inevitable sensory and physiological response to tissue damage: there was little recognition or understanding of the effects on pain perception of individual expectations, anxiety, past experience or genetic differences.[18] Moreover, there was no distinction made between 'acute' and 'chronic' pain states. The legacy of Cicely Saunders and other pioneers in the pain and palliative care fields was to encourage clinicians to see beyond a narrow biomedical perspective on pain and to instead recognise how crucial the subjective experience of pain is. They helped clinicians recognise the difference between acute and chronic pain, showing that the latter persists long after the tissue damage that initially triggered its onset has resolved, and to embrace a wider set of solutions for the relief of pain than was otherwise popular at the time. Contemporary definitions of pain make it clear that pain:

➤ is an individual experience
➤ comprises emotional and sensorial components
➤ has temporal characteristics
➤ has undefined boundaries.[19]

While any detailed discussion of pain is beyond the scope of this chapter, in essence the palliative care approach to pain management, particularly in severe or chronic pain states, involves taking an interdisciplinary approach to integrate the efforts of healthcare providers from several disciplines, each of whom specialises in different features of the pain experience.[18] It also involves the systematic application of up to date clinical techniques to measuring, assessing and relieving pain. To this extent, pain as been recently termed the 'fifth vital sign'.[20] In cancer care, the development of the WHO's 'three step ladder'[21] which provides a simple guide to the use of analgesia in cancer pain and emphasises the importance of regular provision and review of pain relief, is a core aspect of the palliative care armoury.

Enhancing quality of life

In their detailed overview of the issues involved in evaluating quality of life, Kaasa and Loge[22] note that 'quality of life' was cited as one of the main goals of healthcare in ancient Greece. Quality of life is essentially a subjectively defined phenomenon, which is difficult to assess or measure. In spite of this, there have been many attempts to operationalise and quantify quality of life in palliative care research.[22]

Sometimes quality of life has been related to the degree to which a person can live a 'normal' life or engage with the range of activities of daily living,[22] or meet the needs identified in Maslow's needs hierarchy, i.e. biological needs, needs for close relationships, needs for meaningful occupation and the need for change.[23] However, these conceptualisations of quality of life do not fit well with the observation that many people living with quite severe illness, with its associated limitations and disabilities, may report a high quality of life. A more useful model is provided by the 'gap' theory of Calman[24] who argued that quality of life is related to the difference between an individual's expectations and their perception of any given situation. The wider the gap between expectation and perception, the less quality of life a person may have. It is important to remember that individual perceptions of what is a reasonable quality of life can change quite dramatically with changes in illness status: this is known as the 'response shift' phenomenon.[25] In palliative care practice, quality of life assessment is complex and encompasses all aspects of health and social care that people affected by life limiting illness require.

Team working

In the NICE Guidance for improving palliative and supportive care in adults with cancer published in England during 2004, the multidisciplinary team is defined as:

> A group of health and social care professionals from a range of disciplines who meet regularly to discuss and agree plans of treatment and care for people with a particular type of cancer or problem, or in a particular location. It includes primary care teams, site specific cancer teams and specialist palliative care teams.[26]

The Guidance goes on to describe how the teams should seek to ensure effective interpersonal communication within the team and between them and other teams. One important aspect that contributes to the success of team working is that each member has respect and values the roles of other colleagues in the team; that leadership is not necessarily always ascribed to one particular professional group; and that decision making is openly shared, while each member accepts at the same time their professional accountability for the particular role they play within the team.[27]

This is not always easy. Sometimes, stereotypes which we may all hold to a greater or lesser extent can get in the way of good team working. In the field of palliative care, this has been a source of stress which has been well described in the research literature.[28] However, as Speck notes, 'in well functioning teams, protective attitudes to professional status and roles will not play a significant role'.[27] Moreover, in order to work within the framework of palliative care as defined by the WHO, team working is imperative and is the only way to achieve 'early identification and impeccable assessment and treatment of pain and other problems, physical, psychosocial and spiritual'.[14] A commitment to team working is an important aspect of the professional duties of all of the clinical professions which contribute to palliative care.

CHALLENGES FOR PALLIATIVE CARE
Palliative care in long-term conditions
Traditionally (and for historical reasons that were alluded to above) palliative care has been offered mainly to people with advanced cancer. This seems to have reinforced the idea that palliative care is relevant only to the last months or weeks of life. However, it is now widely accepted that there is no sudden movement from, on the one hand, curative care, to, on the other hand, palliative care, especially for people living with long-term conditions. The two styles of care can co-exist over a long period of time, although clearly the emphasis will shift and change according to a person's needs.

One of the problems associated with access to palliative care at an early stage is that of evaluating and encouraging recognition of the value of such an approach, and of knowing when to refer patients for support or to seek advice from specialists in palliative care. Although it is widely agreed in principle that palliative care has an important role to play early in a course of serious illness, in practice care of this type is often delivered late in a person's disease process. The reasons behind this are complex, and may be partly to do with cultural and social attitudes to illness, death and healthcare, and partly due to issues of prognostication. People who have diseases other than cancer may be especially disadvantaged, not because of lack of awareness of palliative care needs on the part of their health providers but because of the uneven and unpredictable course that their illness may follow.

Palliative care in older age
In the developed world, we are all living longer, sometimes well into our 80s and 90s with the result that many more people are living with serious chronic illness and disability towards the end of their lives. Palliative care therefore needs to embrace a much wider range of issues than it has in the past. However, among many older people there may be no definable moment at which 'dying' commences and the complex factors which lead to death can only be understood retrospectively.[29] It is a paradox therefore that it frequently remains the

case that the label of 'dying' is often necessary to open the door to palliative care service provision. In the UK, evidence has been accumulating since the early 1970s which suggests that the experience of living in the last year of life for older people and their carers is marked by extreme disadvantage in terms of health and social care provision, particularly specialist palliative care.[30] These result on the one hand from ageist stereotypes that predominated in the 20th century and which are only now coming under sustained critique,[31] and on the other from entrenched disease focused models of palliative care service delivery, which, while they have served the needs of cancer patients well, have probably been detrimental to the imaginative design of services to meet the complex intersection of health and social needs in the new circumstances in which the last year of life tends to be associated with 'problems caused by great old age and its troubles as well as any final illness'.[32]

Palliative care in resource poor settings

Very few people who have palliative care needs or who are in need of support as they enter the dying phase are cared for in settings which have advantages and resources for care available to hospice and specialist palliative care services, whether inpatient based or in the community – indeed, such care has been described as 'five star care for the few'.[33] This is perhaps most obviously the case in non Western countries where lack of economic resources for any kind of healthcare is a fundamental barrier to the delivery of any non familial health-care to people in need, let alone palliative care. However, it is also true of some environments of care in the developed world. The situation of care homes for older people or those with long-term disabilities, which are outside the NHS and thus have commonly reported[34] problems in accessing support for their residents, is perhaps the clearest example.

There are a number of initiatives directed at providing a 'toolkit' for palliative care in resource poor settings, some of which are aimed at developing countries but from which much can be extrapolated and applied in settings in the developed world that are currently impoverished.[35]

In England, in recognition of a fundamental lack of equity of access to palliative care resources, the End of Life Care Strategy[36] has been developed to inform and guide service development to meet the needs of all those with palliative care needs. The term 'end of life care' has been used to try to break the association made in the minds of many between 'palliative care' and 'cancer care', and to highlight the widespread nature of the need to support people affected by palliative care needs, regardless of their diagnosis or the place in which they are located. The strategy makes clear that the aim is to make:

> a step change in access to high quality care for all people approaching the end of life. This should be irrespective of age, gender, ethnicity, religious belief,

disability, sexual orientation, diagnosis or socioeconomic deprivation. High quality care should be available wherever the person may be: at home, in a care home, in hospital, in a hospice or elsewhere.[37]

As the English End of Life Care Strategy highlights, a number of other countries have also developed, since 2000, work programmes and strategies to improve palliative and end of life care provision. These countries include Australia, Canada and New Zealand. Each country has focused on access, integration of services, outcome measures, research and education, with the ultimate goal of achieving more equitable access to better quality services for all in need.

CONCLUSION

This chapter has outlined how palliative care emerged as a philosophy and mode of practice in the mid 20th century and has led to fundamental changes, some of which remain aspirational, in the care of people affected by life limiting illness. Palliative care operates at the intersection of illness and disease, providing a reminder that a person with disease is socially and biographically located and will have a unique response to their condition and situation. It focuses on enhancing the person's own ability to cope with illness, on strengthening their relationships with others, on helping them to live their remaining life as comfortably as possible and managing pain and symptoms at the end of their life by applying the best skills and knowledge of the multidisciplinary team. In the last few years, the principles of palliative care have been employed to shape policy guidance relating to end of life care at a national and international level, providing an unparalleled opportunity to strategically shape the quality of care for all those in need. From a modality of care reserved for the few, palliative care has been recognised as widely applicable to the many, working in partnership with many other disciplines and models of care.

REFERENCES

1 Sepulveda C, Marlin A, Yoshida T, *et al*. Palliative care: the WHO global perspective. *J Pain Symptom Manage*. 2002; 24(2): 91–6.

2 Clark D, Seymour J. *Reflections on Palliative Care*. Buckingham: Open University Press; 1999.

3 Winslow M, Clark D. *St Joseph's Hospice, Hackney: a century of caring in the East End of London*. Lancaster: Observatory Publications; 2005.

4 Clark D. Cradled to the grave? Terminal care in the United Kingdom, 1946–67. *Mortality*. 1999; 4(3): 225–47.

5 Clark D. 'Total pain', disciplinary power and the body in the work of Cicely Saunders, 1958–1967. *Soc Sci Med*. 1999; 49: 727–36.

6 Seymour JE, Clark D, Winslow M. Pain and palliative care: the emergence of new specialties. *J Pain Symptom Manage*. 2005; 29(1): 2–13.

7 Worcester A. *The Care of the Aged, the Dying and the Dead*. New York: Arno Press; 1977. (Reprint of 1935 original.) p. 48.

8 Kearney M. *A Place of Healing: working with suffering in living and dying*. Oxford: Oxford University Press; 2000.

9 Randall F, Downie R. *The Philosophy of Palliative Care: critique and reconstruction*. Oxford: Oxford University Press; 2006.

10 Clark D. *Cicely Saunders, Founder of the Hospice Movement, Selected Letters 1959–1999*. Oxford: Oxford University Press; 2002.

11 Clark D, Wright M. The International Observatory on End of Life Care: a global view of palliative care development. *J Pain Symptom Manage*. 2007; 33(5): 542–6.

12 Davies E, Higginson I, editors. *The Solid Facts: palliative care*. Copenhagen: WHO; 2004. Available at: www.euro.who.int/document/E82931.pdf (accessed 8 August 2008).

13 World Health Organization. *Definition of Palliative Care*. Available at: www.who.int/cancer/palliative/definition/en/ (accessed 8 August 2008).

14 National Council for Palliative Care. *Changing Gear: guidelines for managing the last days of life in adults*. London: National Council for Palliative Care; 2006, p. 10.

15 Cassell E. *The Nature of Suffering and the Goals of Medicine*. Oxford: Oxford University Press; 2004.

16 Kleinman A. *The Illness Narratives: suffering, healing and the human condition*. New York: Basic Books; 1988.

17 Proudfoot W. Commenting on 'Living with dying', Saunders CM. *Man and Medicine*. 1976; 1: 246. Cited in: Clark D. Total pain: the work of Cicely Saunders and the hospice movement. *American Pain Society Bulletin*. 2000; 10(4). Available at: www.ampainsoc.org/pub/bulletin/jul00/hist1.htm (accessed 10 August 2008).

18 Baszanger I. *Inventing Pain Medicine: from the laboratory to the clinic*. New Brunswick: Rutgers University Press; 1998.

19 Paz S, Seymour JE. Pain: theories, evaluation and management. In: Payne S, Ingleton C, Seymour JE, editors. *Palliative Care Nursing: principles and evidence for practice*. 2nd ed. Buckingham: Open University Press; 2008.

20 Jackson M. *Pain: the fifth vital sign*. New York: Crown Publishers; 2002.

21 World Health Organization. *Expert Committee Report Cancer Pain Relief and Palliative Care*. Technical Report Series 804. Geneva: WHO; 1990.

22 Kaasa S, Loge JH. Quality of life in palliative care: principles and practice. In: Doyle D, Hanks G, Cherny N, *et al.*, editors. *Oxford Textbook of Palliative Medicine*. 3rd ed. Oxford: Oxford University Press; 2004. pp. 196–210.

23 Maslow A. *Motivation and Personality*. New York: Harper; 1970.

24 Calman K. Quality of life in cancer patients: an hypothesis. *J Med Ethics*. 1984; 10(3): 124–7.

25 Sprangers MA, Schwartz CE. Integrating response shift into health-related quality of life research: a theoretical model. *Soc Sci Med*. 1999; 48: 1507–15.

26 National Institute for Health and Clinical Excellence. *Guidance on Cancer Services: improving supportive and palliative care for adults with cancer*. London: NICE; 2004. p. 200.

27 Speck P. *Teamwork in Palliative Care, Fulfilling or Frustrating?* Oxford: Oxford University Press; 2006. p. 194.

28 Vachon M. Occupational stress in palliative care. In: O'Connor M, Aranda S, editors. *Palliative Nursing Care: a guide to practice*. Oxford: Radcliffe Publishing; 2003.

29 Lloyd L. Morality and mortality: ageing and the ethics of care. *Ageing and Society*. 2004; **24**: 235–56.

30 Grande GE, Addington-Hall JM, *et al*. Place of death and access to home care services: are certain patient groups at a disadvantage? *Soc Sci Med*. 1999; 47(5): 565–78.

31 Seymour JE, Witherspoon R, Gott M, *et al*. *End of Life Care: promoting comfort, choice and well being among older people facing death*. Bristol: Policy Press; 2005.

32 Davies E, Higginson I, editors. *Better Palliative Care for Older People*. Copenhagen: WHO; 2004.

33 Field D. Palliative medicine and the medicalization of death. *Eur J Cancer Care*. 1994; **3**(2): 58–62.

34 Froggatt K. *Palliative Care in Care Homes for Older People*. London: National Council for Palliative Care; 2004.

35 Coombes R. Palliative care toolkit developed for staff in developing countries. *BMJ*. 2008; **336**: 913.

36 Department of Health. *End of Life Care Strategy: promoting high quality care for all adults at the end of life*. London: DH; 2008.

37 Department of Health, op. cit. para. 7.

CHAPTER 3

Supportive and palliative care needs in progressive long-term neurological conditions: an overview

Jane Seymour and Penny McNamara

This chapter provides an overview of the supportive and palliative care needs and problems experienced by people with a progressive long-term neurological condition (PLTNC) and those friends and family members who provide daily care and support to them. As noted in the introduction, in this book our focus is on the four most common progressive conditions: motor neurone disease, Parkinson's disease, multiple sclerosis and Huntington's disease, but there are many other conditions[1] giving rise to both similar and contrasting needs which come under the umbrella of PLTNCs. This chapter draws together a selected range of relevant international evidence relating to palliative and end of life care in PLTNCs but readers need to be aware that a fully systematic review of the literature is beyond our scope. In particular, we draw readers' attention to guidelines that have recently become available as a result of a programme of work conducted under the auspices of the National Council for Palliative Care in England examining the interfaces of palliative, rehabilitative and neurological care across a number of PLTNCs.[2] Before looking at the latter guidelines and reviewing some the evidence that underpins them, we provide a sketch of some key epidemiological features and also briefly explain some policy developments occurring in the UK that are of relevance to those affected by PLTNCs and other chronic diseases.

AN EPIDEMIOLOGICAL SKETCH

Chronic illness has now become the most common route to death in the UK; over 15 million people in England have long-term health needs as a result of such conditions.[3] The numbers of those with such needs will rise with increasing longevity. Chronic illnesses are classically longstanding or recurrent with no cure. They are not always progressive and not usually immediately life threatening, but when they do progress they may ultimately shorten the life of the person with the condition. We have an ageing population, with the number of people over the age of 85 projected to rise by approximately 75% by 2025.[3] With a greater number of people living longer with chronic disease, the impact on the healthcare system is extensive. It has been estimated that the care of people with chronic needs demands over two thirds of NHS activity and an estimated 80% of its costs.[2] Chronic diseases in their entirety were responsible for 75% (389 431) of all deaths in England and Wales in 2005.[4] Circulatory diseases (including heart disease and stroke) have been the most common causes of death in England and Wales during the last 90 years, followed by cancer and respiratory disease. The progress report issued by the NHS End of Life Care Programme[5] calculates that neurological conditions were the primary cause of 14 606 deaths in England during 2004 – just 2.8% of the overall deaths. However death rates may provide limited indication of the real burden of suffering caused by neurological conditions as death registrations do not always recognise the presence of any underlying disease when it is not seen to be the immediate cause of death. For instance, pneumonia may be indicated as the immediate cause of death with aspiration as a cause for that. The underlying medical condition may not be mentioned on the death certificate in spite of guidance encouraging medical practitioners to be as comprehensive as possible when considering a cause of death.

The NHS Healthcare Workforce[6] highlights that:

➤ approximately 10 million people across the UK have a PLTNC, accounting for 20% of acute hospital admissions
➤ 350 000 people in the UK need help with the activities of daily living because of a neurological condition
➤ 850 000 people care for someone with a neurological condition.

The needs of those affected are complex and variable, with fundamental impacts on daily life, often over many years, and a fluctuating but inexorable movement from requirements for low level support to needs for continuous palliative care focused support towards the end of life. The National Council for Palliative Care[7] notes a number of major differences in the supportive and palliative care needs of people with neurological conditions as compared to the 'typical' case where needs arise from cancer.

➤ In most cases, PLTNCs have a longer and more variable time course.
➤ Most PLTNCs are prone to relapse and remission and, as a consequence, it is often difficult to know when the person affected is in their final stages of life.

➤ Symptoms related to PLTNCs are diverse and complex and often accompanied by disabilities including cognitive, behavioural and communication problems, as well as physical problems such as pain and various forms of disablement.

POLICY: CONTEXT AND CHALLENGES IN THE UK

As discussed in the previous chapter, in the UK specialised palliative care tends to be provided mainly to people with advanced cancer, and historically its provision has been uneven around the country.[8] This is in spite of evidence that those who die of non-malignant diseases have as many complex care needs (thus potentially requiring specialist palliative care provision) as those with advanced cancer.[9] There have been a number of policy developments addressing this problem. In particular, there has been a trend towards emphasising the value of attending to general palliative care principles, and applying these in all conditions and in all settings, rather than focusing solely on extending specialist palliative care. The National Council for Palliative Care (previously the National Council for Hospice and Specialist Palliative Care Services) states that the principles of general palliative care include the following:

➤ a focus on quality of life
➤ a 'whole person' approach
➤ care which encompasses both the person who is ill and those who are important to that person
➤ respect for choice and autonomy
➤ emphasis on open communication.

The National Service Framework for Long-term (Neurological) Conditions[10] provides Quality Requirements for services delivered to people living with PLTNCs that are cognisant of these principles. Quality Requirement 9 in the document proposes that people with PLTNCs receive 'a comprehensive range of palliative care services when they need them' and that these services should meet their needs for 'personal, social psychological and spiritual support, in line with the principles of palliative care' ([10:5]).

However, there is little understanding of how organisations can integrate their services with those of other providers effectively to achieve this 'comprehensive range' or what the challenges are facing service providers in so doing. Authorities responsible for service commissioning authorities have been reported as having both little awareness of the needs of people with PLTNCs, and a lack of knowledge about the incidence and prevalence of the conditions in their localities, which creates a significant constraint.[11] Other policy and service organisation challenges identified in a review of the literature relate to: problems in creating multidisciplinary teams; the use of specialist nurses/key workers;

'health' and 'social' care boundaries and the under recognition of the potential for self managed care.[12] The End of Life Strategy for England[13] highlights the need for organisations to attend to these issues in order to maximise the quality of support and experience for people, such as those living with PLTNCs, who have complex needs across the life course. It depicts an end of life care pathway that involves the following steps.

➤ Identification of people approaching the end of life and initiating discussions about preferences for end of life care.

➤ Care planning: assessing needs and preferences, agreeing a care plan to reflect these and reviewing these regularly.

➤ Coordination of care.

➤ Delivery of high quality services in all locations.

➤ Management of the last days of life.

➤ Care after death.

➤ Support for carers, both during a person's illness and after their death.

SUPPORTIVE AND PALLIATIVE CARE NEEDS: A REVIEW OF THE EVIDENCE

Supportive and palliative care needs among people with PLTNCs may be present from diagnosis but the long length of the disease trajectory in some conditions – people with multiple sclerosis, Parkinson's disease and Huntington's disease may live for as many as 15 to 25 years after diagnosis – means that it can be difficult to judge when to introduce an approach which focuses on palliative care principles as opposed to more narrowly disease focused management.[14] In contrast, people with motor neurone disease may live for only a few months, with very rapid deterioration posing challenges for supportive and palliative care management that require urgent attention. In all cases, patients may require intensive input from rehabilitation and therapy teams at the same time as symptom management and supportive non clinical care. PLTNCs are characterised by a loss of motor, sensory and cognitive functions, which results in gradually increasing disability and dependence.[15] Beyond this obvious commonality surrounding key characteristics of disease progression, people with PLTNCs have a great diversity of needs. For example, symptoms related to different conditions and within conditions vary greatly and each person will, over time, experience many different symptoms. Some of these will recur frequently while others will disappear partially or completely, only to be replaced by a different symptom or group of symptoms. This makes long-term care planning difficult. People with advanced disease as a result of PLTNCs present a range of problems which may make both care delivery and advance planning for care in the last stages of life both complex and challenging: ethically, practically and clinically. This is due to the range of physical, cognitive and emotional problems that are experienced towards the end of life as well as issues of communication, decision making about nutrition and technologies of life support, and family care.[16]

Motor neurone disease

Motor neurone disease (MND) is a rare, progressive and often rapidly fatal disorder, which involves degeneration of the motor system at all levels.[17] Its cause, except for developing knowledge about the role of genetic influences that have been identified in some rare familial forms, is unknown.[15] It leads to paralysis of the cranial and skeletal muscles and has been described as characterised by a series of losses to not only the person with the devastating condition but also those close to that person.[18,19] In most cases, the person with the disease remains intellectually intact until death, but subject to progressive immobility and requiring care for every aspect of their needs. People with MND have been reported as experiencing an existential 'crisis' characterised by a pervasive loss of control of all aspects of their lives: bodily, social and communicative, and involving a struggle to learn how to accept care from others.[18]

Approximately half of patients affected die within three years of diagnosis,[17] some doing so within months rather than years. Some people present with what is known as 'bulbar onset' that involves slurring of speech (dysarthria), difficulty swallowing (dysphagia), or both. Other patients may present with upper or lower limb weakness. Bulbar onset, together with older age and low forced respiratory capacity, tends to indicate a poorer prognosis.[17] Commonly occurring symptoms experienced by people living with MND are detailed in Box 3.1.

BOX 3.1 Symptoms of MND

- Weakness and atrophy
- Fasciculation and muscle cramps
- Spasticity
- Dysarthria
- Dysphagia and drooling
- Dyspnoea
- Pathological laughter or tearfulness
- Psychic disturbances
- Sleep disturbances
- Pain
- Thick mucous secretions
- Hypoventilation
- Constipation

Source:[17,20]

People with MND may, by the time they receive their diagnosis (which can take many months from recognition by the person of the first signs of illness), be distrustful of clinicians (in those instances where they have been searching for an explanation about their problems) and extremely frightened by their symptoms. The communication of the diagnosis is therefore a pivotal moment in the palliative care trajectory of patients with MND, since it will set the tone of the relationship between the clinical team, the patient and the family. We examine issues of diagnostic disclosure and communication below.

Multiple sclerosis

Multiple sclerosis (MS) is the most common demyelinating disease, i.e. involving the myelin covering of nervous tissue. It commonly has an unpredictable, relapsing and remitting course followed by progressive deterioration prior to a terminal stage, with each relapse tending to be followed by an incomplete recovery.[21] It is the commonest cause of neurological disability in young adults and is more common in women than in men. As in MND, its causes are largely unknown, although some genetic and environmental factors are implicated.[21] Lesions which result from MS can be widely scattered throughout the nervous system and give rise to a variety of symptoms, signs and problems in people affected by the disease. Everyone with the disease will suffer a gradual escalation in disease burden involving problems with weakness, spasticity, tremor, loss of mobility, fatigue, visual loss and urinary symptoms. In some people, swallowing difficulties may also be present and many people suffer from pain, the severity of which relates to the degree of demyelination. A minority of people suffer from disorders of emotional expression, which can result in a lack of ability to control emotions or expression of emotions that do not mirror how the person feels subjectively. Many people will experience severe challenges coping with symptoms that are somewhat 'hidden' from others: fatigue is a common problem of this type.[22] Fifteen years post diagnosis, between one third and two thirds of people need to use a support for walking, most will have had to give up paid work, and a minority will be bedridden.[21] As for people with MND, although experienced over a longer period of time, losses are incremental and relentless for people with MS and those to whom they are close. As we shall see with Parkinson's disease, death occurs in people with MS as a result of an associated infection or as a result of a co-morbid condition such as heart disease.

Parkinson's disease

Parkinson's disease (PD) is a common progressive PLTNC disease that is estimated to affect one on 500 people in the UK population,[23] with a prevalence that increases with age. The neuropathology of the disease is related to the depletion of dopamine producing cells which gives rise to the well recognised motor symptoms of the disease: resting tremor, rigidity and bradykinesia.[24] Non motor symptoms, such as depression and anxiety, sleep disturbances, autonomic dysfunction (causing, for example, urinary symptoms or impotence) and variable pain syndromes, occur across the course of the disease, also causing disability and significant long-term distress.[24] The disease progresses in stages from early, moderate and then advanced phases, with the advanced phase tending to be protracted.[19] The advanced stage has been defined[23] as being characterised by the experience of two or more of the following clinical and quality or life related symptoms:

➤ drug treatment no longer effective
➤ drug regimes increasingly complex
➤ 'off' periods
➤ dyskinesias
➤ mobility problems and falls
➤ swallowing problems
➤ psychiatric signs (depression, anxiety, hallucinations, psychosis)
➤ reduced independence
➤ less control and predictability in the overall disease picture.

In PD death usually occurs as a result of an associated infection or from a co-morbid condition, rather than as a direct result of the disease itself.[23]

Huntington's disease

Huntington's disease (HD) is a genetically inherited condition leading to progressive deterioration of physical, cognitive and emotional states so that the affected individual becomes profoundly incapacitated. Each child of an affected parent has a 50% chance of disease inheritance. Although HD can appear in childhood, it is generally described as a late onset disease that usually occurs in mid adulthood. However clear appearance of disease signs and symptoms can be preceded by minor abnormalities (such as restlessness), which may have been present for many years.[25,26] Death usually occurs between 10 and 20 years after the clear onset of symptoms and, similarly to PD and MS, is usually precipitated by secondary infection. The disease is characterised by progressive dementia and characteristic involuntary movements known as 'chorea', together with behaviour abnormalities. The latter include outbursts of apparently angry or aggressive behaviours that are difficult for caregivers to predict and to deal with and may, for some, be associated with a criminal record.[26] In contrast, at other times, people with HD may suffer from periods of apparent apathy or disinterest in their surroundings, or have hidden depression. Rates of suicide are about four times higher in people with HD than among the general population. HD is recognised to be one of the most devastating of conditions, not least because of its familial character. Family caregivers are often profoundly involved in care giving to the person with HD, while potentially facing future encounters with the disease.

DIAGNOSTIC DISCLOSURE: ESTABLISHING A PALLIATIVE CARE APPROACH TO COMMUNICATION IN PLTNCs

Receiving news of the diagnosis of a PLTNC is always going to be difficult and stressful, for both the person with the disease and their relatives or partners. The fields of palliative care and communication practice have together developed principles of breaking bad news which are well described in the literature (*see* for example[27,28]) and which, if done well, create the foundation upon which the future palliative care of the patient and the family can be successfully based.

➤ Preparation: find out from the patient as early as possible whether they are the sort of person who likes to know detailed information, and whether they would wish a family member to be with them when any information about their illness is given to them.

➤ Get the environment right: finding a place where it is possible to sit in comfort and privacy is essential.

➤ Giving a warning shot: rather than immediately launching into a detailed explanation, it is often better to warn that you have some news that may not be good, e.g. 'We have your test results back and they are not as good as we had hoped.'

➤ Find out how much the patient wishes to know and what they already understand about their illness.

➤ Allow time for the patient and family to express their feelings.

➤ Plan with the patient and their family member(s) what will happen next and ensure that they feel supported.

In disclosing a diagnosis of a PLTNC, a key challenge for the clinical team is to establish a trusting relationship in which open communication is engendered, and to provide information and help to the patient and their family as their needs unfold at a pace which is dictated by the patient and yet which is carefully and proactively planned so that major crises are avoided. Privacy, willingness to listen, lack of interruptions and a warm, empathic manner are essential if the encounter is to be helpful to patients and their families. Drawing on experience of diagnostic disclosure with patients with MND ([29:34]), Sloan and colleagues recommend that clinicians consider three underlying objectives.

1 Do not withhold information if the patient wants it.
2 Do not impose information if the patient does not want it.
3 Gauge and respond to the patient's reaction to the news.

Here, important differences among patients may become clear, which can be related to cultural or ethnic background as well as social class and educational or religious beliefs. One size will not fit all, which makes this a challenging area of practice for clinicians.

The diagnostic encounter is likely to set the scene for later consultations that will, in some cases, have far reaching impacts on the ability of the whole family to deal with the losses and dilemmas associated with PLTNCs. This is especially the case in HD. Its familial nature means that diagnostic disclosure will have far reaching impacts on the wider family; in many cases, families will be trying to deal with the onset of the disease in a parent while trying to make difficult decisions about testing of children. Where families are affected by divorce or separation, this may make such situations potentially even more difficult.

O'Brien[15] reports on research,[30] which examined the experience of 50 patients who had recently received a diagnosis of MND: most patients could identify positive elements in the disclosure of their diagnosis, since it provided an explanation for their problems and symptoms. Most preferred the diagnosis to be given in a fairly direct yet empathic way, with someone to whom they were close present. For people affected by MND, once their diagnosis is confirmed, some may admit to fear of the process of dying and in particular the risk of 'choking' to death. It has been recommended[17] that these individuals and those whose forced vital capacity drops below 50% should be offered information about the terminal phase, describing the typical last stages of life which for most people involve coma and peaceful death. We examine issues of advance care planning and the management of the last days of life in relation to all PLTNCs below.

In all cases, people affected by a PLTNC will wish to have a source of reliable support and information that they can access once they return home. Providing too much information at the time of diagnosis is, for many people, a source of stress. However, equally, not knowing where to source help with the inevitable questions, fears and concerns that will arise following diagnosis will negatively impact on people's abilities to cope with their condition and be a cause of significant distress. The role of disease associations (such as the Huntington's Disease Association or the Motor Neurone Disease Association) is extremely important since they are repositories of well written information and tried and tested advice on accessing help, as is the role of key workers such as clinical nurse specialists who can follow patients up once they return home. The continuity of care afforded by such key workers is extremely highly valued by people with PLTNCs and their families and will be a key means of providing post diagnostic and long-term support.

CASE EXAMPLE 3.1 Charles

Charles was 46 when he was diagnosed with MND. He presented with weakness in his dominant arm. He remembers being told his diagnosis and the shock he experienced in the next few days. He looks back and describes it like a time just after someone you care about has died. He was emotionally very labile and preoccupied with thoughts of the future and of memories of the past and thinking he would never do certain things again. He lives alone and for the first 18 months after diagnosis he managed to look after himself without any additional care. He gradually lost more power in his arms and lost a considerable amount of weight as it took so long to prepare and eat meals. He became unable to speak and texted his family and friends as a means of communicating to them. It was when this and the whole effort of looking after himself became more difficult that he tried to take his life with an overdose of sleeping tablets. This resulted in a hospital admission and psychological assessment. During the admission he decided that rather than expedite his death he wanted more active management and more support. He requested and had inserted a percutaneous endoscopic gastrostomy (PEG) tube, something he had previously declined. He returned home and the hospital admission triggered a series of healthcare professionals to assess his needs or to reassess them. He had input from the occupational therapist, physiotherapist, dietician and palliative care team in addition to the district nurses. Some months later he decided that he was no longer able to cope on his own and felt unable to deal with the fears that overwhelmed him when he was alone. These fears were disclosed during conversations exploring his wishes regarding future care, as part of advanced care planning. His initial assessment for long-term nursing home care was not supported by the local authority responsible for continuing care funding, but on appeal and in view of his predicted deterioration, this was granted.

PSYCHOSOCIAL NEEDS IN PLTNCs: MAINTAINING DIGNITY AND MEANING

The disclosure of the diagnosis of a PLTNC is the first step in a long trajectory of unfolding needs for psychosocial support and accompaniment that people affected by such conditions will experience.[31] Proving psychosocial support involves the helping of patients and their families to come to terms in their own unique way with what is happening and to assist them in finding the resources and strategies to manage their difficulties, and maintain a sense of meaning and dignity. It also involves addressing issues of loss and grief, fear and the range of other spiritual, emotional and social elements that are associated with life limiting illness.[31] Getting psychosocial support right can have major positive impacts on the well-being of the whole family unit which extend far into bereavement.[32] However, the psychosocial aspects of PLTNCs have, on the whole, been little researched.[33] In the field of MND, it has been shown that where psychosocial needs are met, people with the disease are better able to adjust to their condition, are less likely to suffer from depression and will have better quality of life scores, even where factors such as age and disease severity are controlled ([34] cited in [33]). Where psychosocial needs are not met, experiences of suffering, fear, hopelessness and desires for hastened death have been shown to be more likely.[35-7] A need for a sense of hope is well documented among patients with all life limiting conditions and their families, although this will often take the form of searching or being able to find meaning in life and in establishing some spiritual identity or connection through the experience of illness or in stoically maintaining a positive outlook in the face of great adversity ([38] cited in [33]).[18,39]

Meeting psychosocial needs involves key workers (who may be nurses, social workers, psychologists or medical practitioners working solely or often in the context of a multidisciplinary team) who have the skills to work with complex and sometimes challenging family dynamics, and with the ability to help patients and families adjust to their changing circumstances and relationships, and gradually assist them to discuss and make important choices about ongoing care planning, particularly when end of life needs begin to come into the frame. At the core of psychosocial support is the ability to be a good communicator. As well as skills of listening, of expressing genuine interest and concern, and of empathy, professionals responsible for communicating with patients and their families need to nurture particular attitudes and values such as: being non judgemental; regarding patients/family members as partners; and respecting the rights of patients to be self determining according to their capacity to do so ([28:16]). Some of these are, at first sight, related to the skills that a trained counsellor may provide but clearly it is neither necessary nor possible for all patients to see a counsellor; all professionals need to develop some basic counselling skills that they can draw upon.

In their overview of psychosocial care of people affected by MND, Gallager and Monroe ([31:147]) highlight the importance of conducting a careful assessment (which may unfold over a number of encounters) of each patient and family, with attention paid to the following:
➤ an understanding of the individual patient;
➤ the effect of the illness of family roles and relationships;
➤ personal histories of family members;
➤ family life cycle issues and how these have been perceived;
➤ previous illness or other crises within the family and how these were handled;
➤ other vulnerable individuals in the family;
➤ the family's physical and social resources.

A key challenge in conducting such assessments will surround how the different perspectives that patients and their close relatives may have are balanced by the listener, and an awareness that stories about family events are dynamic 'living' narratives in which the ways they are recounted are often just as important as the nature of the 'facts' contained therein. Moreover, views and deeply held convictions can change quite rapidly with time, and good psychosocial care needs to take the form of recurrent reviews of plans, particularly where a patient's condition involves rapid change and deterioration. Sometimes the resolution of profoundly difficult practical and ethical dilemmas can only take place in the situated context of the family history and biography, understanding of which has to be founded on the development over weeks, months and years of a close relationship between the key worker(s), patient and family. Research among people with HD and their family carers has clearly demonstrated the importance of 'care co-coordinators' (who do not necessarily need to have a clinical background) who can provide information, help with access to supportive services, provide emotional and moral support and assess, review and evaluate ongoing plans for care.[26]

FAMILY CARERS' NEEDS

While inextricably linked to the issue of psychosocial support, it is worth specifically noting how critical issues of supporting family carers are, both during the course of PLTNCs and after bereavement. PLTNCs are all associated with significant needs for care, a role often fulfilled by close family members whose needs may sometimes be subsumed to those of the person receiving care. In an Australian national survey which elicited responses from 503 people with the four PLTNCs that are the focus of this chapter, and from 373 carers,[19] extensive unmet needs for support were found, with patients and carers in the HD and MND groups reporting the highest needs. People with MS were less likely than any other group to have a carer to provide daily care, and patients and carers in the HD and PD groups were most likely to report depression and anxiety. People with MND were almost twice as likely as other respondents to report that their informal carer had given up work in order to provide care, and they and their carers also reported a poor quality of life and satisfaction with quality of life equivalent to that reported by those with HD. MND carers reported the lowest quality of life across all four groups, largely because of 'fatigue and tiredness' ([19:375]). Such findings are likely to be related to the unrelenting nature and physical hard work involved in caring for someone who becomes rapidly physically disabled, as well as the associated sadness and profound distress such an experience is associated with.[40] In the case of all PLTNCs, carers have to become used to negotiating the total care of the ill person's body: managing intimate personal and bodily needs that some may find challenging and uncomfortable to cope with and which, in our society, are sometimes seen as stigmatising and shameful. If carers are to cope and deal well with their subsequent bereavement, they need high quality respite care that is acceptable to them and to the patient, as well as information about affordable and accessible social and practical help, and financial assistance.

KEY PRINCIPLES IN PAIN CONTROL IN PLTNCs

Only a brief and general overview will be provided here of this issue, since it is covered in Chapter 4 in some detail. It is beyond the scope of this chapter to look at the wide range of other symptoms that patients with PLTNC suffer; readers are again directed to Chapter 4 for consideration of these, and to a number of specialist texts which deal with this issue.

Pain, as noted above, is a feature in all PLTNCs and is common in MS and in MND, with up to 50% and 75% of patients suffering in the respective conditions: this is an incidence which is higher than in some cancers. Pain may have many causes, but is often neuropathic or muscular in origin. Neuropathic pain is that which results from damage to the nervous system, such a peripheral nerve, the dorsal root ganglion or dorsal root, or the central nervous system.[41] It is only in recent years that pain has been acknowledged as a significant problem in PLTNCs, perhaps mirroring a change in clinical practice as a result of the widespread acceptance that pain is 'whatever the experiencing person says it is, existing whenever he says it does' ([42:95] cited in [43]) or as 'what the patient says hurts' ([44:17]). These three 'classic' definitions present pain as:

➤ being an individual experience
➤ comprising emotional and sensorial components
➤ having temporal characteristics
➤ having undefined boundaries.

In PLTNCs most pain is of the chronic form, differing from acute pain which is a normal sensation triggered in the nervous system by tissue damage. Chronic pain is persistent after tissue healing or may occur in the absence of tissue damage. It is related to complex underlying neurological dysfunction and is often difficult to completely eradicate using drugs alone. Such pain requires a complex and multidimensional approach to its treatment and tends to have a more profound impact on a patient's general well-being than acute pain: it often affects a person's mood, personality and social relationships. There is also a synergy between the experience of pain and the meanings that the person in pain associates with it. For example, if the experience of pain is associated by the patient with fear of increasing disability or fear of an unknown feature, their pain is likely to be more difficult to treat and may gradually become more and more severe. People with chronic pain usually experience concomitant depression, sleep disturbance, fatigue and decreased overall physical and mental functioning.[45] Treatment of chronic pain, particularly of the neuropathic variety, may require a mixture of pharmacological and non pharmacological strategies. Some patients may find complementary or alternative treatments such as reflexology or massage very helpful. Where pharmacological treatment is required, this should initially be provided in line with the World Health Organization (WHO) framework of the 'three step analgesic ladder'.[45] The three step ladder is the method most widely accepted and recognised as the basis for adequate and safe pain control. Its methodology involves a stepwise approach to the use of analgesic drugs, going from the first (simple non opioid analgesics and any necessary adjuvants) through the use of weak opioids and any required adjuvants, to the third step, which involves strong opioids which are carefully titrated upwards until pain is relieved, again with the use of adjuvants as required. Key associated aspects of the recommendations made by the WHO are that pain relief should, where possible, be administered orally, at regular intervals and subject to regular review. The right dose and combination of analgesic therapy is that which relieves pain in the individual patient.

MANAGING AND PLANNING FOR END OF LIFE CARE IN PLTNCs

In people with MND, death will usually occur as a result of respiratory failure, while in the other conditions, death is often as a result of an associated infection precipitated by the weakness and frailty of progressive disease.

In MND, respiratory failure can occur quite quickly and, as a result, death may sometimes happen relatively suddenly.[47] This means that it is imperative that decisions have been made in advance of respiratory deterioration about what action, if any, the patient and family wish to take in the event of respiratory failure. With the onset of new technologies such as non invasive ventilation and percutaneous endoscopic gastrostomy (PEG) feeding, the terminal course of MND can be delayed for significant periods of time, although the character of the terminal course is little affected by such interventions.[47] While for many patients, interventions such as these may enable precious days, weeks or months of life, they are not necessarily the right choice for all. Sensitive advance care planning discussions which may need to take place over many weeks or months are necessary in order to inform what is in the patient's best interests in advance of the terminal phase.

Some patients may feel very strongly that they do not wish to receive technological support at the end of life, since this is merely delaying the inevitable. In these cases they may, once the clinician caring for them is satisfied that they have had appropriate information and can weigh up and retain the implications of the latter, wish to draft an advance decision to refuse life prolonging treatment.[48] These, where they are assessed as valid and applicable, have legal force under the Mental Capacity Act of 2005. In all cases, providing sensitive information in a staged fashion about the process of dying can lay to rest very significant fears among patients and families. For example, many with MND fear choking to death but these fears have been shown from a number of research studies to be largely unfounded.[47] The role of opioids in relieving symptoms should be carefully explained to patients and relatives, against a background of research which shows that where opioids such as morphine are used according to standards of best practice and evidence, they do not hasten death and can be used in increasing doses, along with appropriate adjuvant therapies, so that pain and other symptoms are well controlled (*see* for example [44]). Typical medications used at the end of life are summarised in Box 3.2.

BOX 3.2 Medications used in the last days of life

- Analgesics – to relieve pain, e.g. morphine
- Anxiolytics/sedatives – to relieve distress and breathlessness, e.g. midazolam
- Anti-secretories – to relieve respiratory tract secretions, e.g. hyoscine hydrobromide
- Anti-emetics – to relieve nausea and vomiting, e.g. cyclizine

(For further details *see* [48:12].)

Some patients may have particular problems that require intervention either by their regular healthcare providers or by referral to specialists. Spiritual distress may be one example. Sykes[47] notes that, in preparing for the end of life, it is only patients that can resolve how best to address their suffering as they approach the end of life and it is the role of nursing, medical and other interventions to help the person find these, not to dictate a particular path for the individual to follow. A particular challenge in PLTNCs is the loss of communication abilities in many patients; this is particularly the case with MND and with HD. The extent of disability for such individuals is such that it is hard, if not impossible, to truly enter their lived experiences. However, staying with patients, attending rigorously and patiently to difficult pain and other symptom related problems, and seeking creative solutions to these, will make end of life care easier for all concerned. Good end of life care requires the clinical team to work together to critically assess the aims and goals of care and treatment in the context of the particular person and his family. Asking questions such as 'Why are we doing this?' or 'What do we hope to achieve from this particular path or therapy?' may enable the multidisciplinary team to act in a manner which is more closely aligned to the person's best interests and less dictated by the biomedical imperative or habits of clinical routine. The overarching aim of all care and treatment at the end of life is to respond quickly and efficiently to the needs that patients and their companions may have, so that their comfort and quality of life is maximised as far as possible. Key principles which underpin the management of end of life care in all conditions are listed in Box 3.3.

BOX 3.3 Key principles in the management of end of life care

- Current medications are assessed and non essentials discontinued.
- 'As required' subcutaneous medication is prescribed according to an agreed protocol to manage pain, agitation, nausea and vomiting and respiratory tract secretions.
- Decisions are taken to discontinue inappropriate interventions, including blood tests, intravenous fluids and observation of vital signs.
- The patient, family and carers are able to communicate in their preferred language.
- The insights of the patient, family and carers into the patient's condition are identified.
- Religious and spiritual needs of the patient, family and carers are assessed.
- Means of informing family and carers of the patient's impending death are identified.
- The family and carers are given appropriate written information.
- The GP practice is made aware of the patient's condition.
- A plan of care is explained and discussed, as far as possible, with the patient and with their family or other carers.

Adapted from:[50]

SUMMARY AND CONCLUSION

In this chapter we have demonstrated the enormous burden of chronic illness on the population. With an increasing life expectancy the years during which chronic illness impacts on health and social care services also increase. Those with PLTNCs face increasing disability and experience symptoms as disparate and as severe as those suffering with cancer. However, the variation in the natural course of these diseases poses problems for healthcare professionals as the triggers to referring into palliative care services are often not as obvious as in the pathway for cancer patients. Furthermore, the length of time a person may live with considerable disability due to advanced disease is often much longer than for patients with cancer. National policy to support the needs of these patients has been published but services providing that support are not yet well established nor integrated into the care pathway these patients find themselves on. National standards and recent policy seek to redress such inequity. Tools such as the Liverpool Care Pathway for the Dying Patient have been employed in generalist settings, and encourage recognition, assessment and management of symptoms in the dying patient and are not disease specific. Those involved in the care of people with PLTNCs need the ongoing support of those more experienced in the use of such tools for them to become part of their routine practice.

REFERENCES

1 Voltz R, Bernat JL, Borasio GD, *et al.*, editors. *Palliative Care in Neurology.* Oxford: Oxford University Press; 2004.

2 Turner-Stokes L, Sykes N, Silber E. Long-term neurological conditions: management at the interface between neurology, rehabilitation and palliative care. *Clin Med.* 2008; 8(2): 186–91.

3 Department of Health. *White Paper: Our Health, Our Care, Our Say: a new direction for community services.* London: COI; 2006.

4 Office of National Statistics. *Mortality statistics.* London: ONS; 2005.

5 Department of Health. *NHS End of Life Care Programme: progress report.* London: DH; 2006.

6 NHS Healthcare Workforce. *Long-term Neurological Conditions: a good practice guide to the development of the multidisciplinary team and the value of the specialist nurses.* London: NHS Healthcare Workforce; 2005. Available at www.healthcareworkforce.nhs.uk/ resources/latest_resources/long_term_neurological_conditions.html (accessed 17 October 2008).

7 National Council for Palliative Care and Royal College of Nursing. *Exploring the Interface: a survey of neurology nurses' involvement with specialist palliative care services and identification of their training needs.* London: NCPC; 2008.

8 National Council for Hospice and Specialist Palliative Care Services. *Palliative Care 2000: commissioning through partnership.* London: NCHSPCS; 1999.

9 Addington-Hall J, Fakhoury W, McCarthy M. Specialist palliative care in non-malignant disease. *Palliat Med.* 1998; 12(6): 417–27.

10 Department of Health. *The National Service Framework for Long-term (Neurological) Conditions.* London: COI; 2005.

11 Sue Ryder Care. *Filling the Void: how real life health information builds better services.* London: Sue Ryder Care; 2007.

12 Wilson E, Elkan R, Seymour J, *et al.* A UK literature review of progressive long-term neurological conditions. *Br J Community Nurs.* 2008; 13(5): 206–12.

13 Department of Health. *End of Life Care Strategy: promoting high quality care for all adults at end of life.* London: DH; 2008.

14 Wollin J, Yates P, Kristjanson L. Supportive and palliative care needs identified by multiple sclerosis patients and their families. *Int J Palliat Nurs.* 2006; 12(1): 20–6.

15 O'Brien T. Neurodegenerative disease. In: Addington-Hall J, Higginson I, editors. *Palliative Care for Non-Cancer Patients.* Oxford: Oxford University Press; 2001. pp. 44–53.

16 Huntington's Disease Society of America. *A Caregiver's Handbook for Advanced Stage Huntington's Disease.* New York: HDSA; 1999.

17 Mitchell JD, Borasio GD. Amyotrophic lateral sclerosis. *Lancet.* 2007; **369**(9578): 2031–41.

18 Brown J. User, carer and professional experiences of care in motor neurone disease. *Primary Health Care Research and Development.* 2003; **4**: 207–17.

19 Kristjanson LJ, Aoun SM, Oldham L. Palliative care and support for people with neurodegenerative conditions and their carers. *Int J Palliat Nurs.* 2005; **12**(8): 368–77.

20 Borasio GD, Voltz R. Palliative care in amyotrophic lateral sclerosis. *J Neurol.* 1997; **224**(Suppl. 4): S11–17.

21 Macleod A, Formaglio F. Demyelinating disease. In: Voltz R, *et al.*, editors. *Palliative Care in Neurology.* Oxford: Oxford University Press; 2004. pp. 27–36.

22 Multiple Sclerosis Society. *MS and Palliative Care: a guide for health and social care professionals.* London: MSS; 2006.

23 Parkinson's Disease Society. *Palliative Care and Advanced Stage Parkinson's Disease.* London: PDS; 2005.

24 Bunting-Perry LK. Palliative care in Parkinson's disease: implications for neuroscience nursing. *J Neurosci Nurs.* 2006; **38**(2): 106–13.

25 Aubeeluck A, Wilson E. Huntington's disease. Part 1: essential background and management. *Br J Nurs.* 2008; **17**(3): 146–51.

26 Dawson S, *et al.* Living with Huntington's disease: needs for supportive care. *Nurs Health Sci.* 2004; **6**: 123–30.

27 Buckman R. Doctors can improve on the way they deliver bad news, MD maintains. Interview by Evelyne Michaels. *CMAJ.* 1992; **146**(4): 564–6.

28 Sheldon F. Communication. In: Sykes N, Edmonds P, Wiles J, editors. *Management of Advanced Disease.* London: Hodder Arnold; 2004. pp. 9–26.

29 Sloan R, Pongratz D, Borasio GD. Communication: breaking bad news. In: Oliver D, Borasio GD, Walsh D, editors. *Palliative Care in Amyotrophic Lateral Sclerosis.* Oxford: Oxford University Press; 2006. pp. 27–42.

30 Johnston M, *et al.* Communicating the diagnosis of motor neurone disease. *Palliat Med.* 1996; **10**(1): 23–34.

31 Gallagher D, Monroe B. Psychosocial care. In: Oliver D, Borasio GD, Walsh D, editors. *Palliative Care in Amyotrophic Lateral Sclerosis.* Oxford: Oxford University Press; 2006. pp. 143–68.

32 Kristjanson L, Toye C, Dawson S. New dimensions in palliative care: a palliative approach to neurodegenerative disease and final illness in older people. *Med J Aust.* 2003; **179**(Suppl.): S41–3.

33 McLeod JE, Clarke DM. A review of psychosocial aspects of motor neurone disease. *J Neurol Sci.* 2007; **258**(1–2): 4–10.

34 McDonald E, *et al.* Survival in amyotrophic lateral sclerosis: the role of psychological factors. *Arch Neurol.* 1994; **51**: 17–23.

35 Ganzini L, Johnston W, Hoffman W. Correlates of suffering in amyotrophic lateral sclerosis. *Neurol.* 1999; **52**: 1434–40.

36 Beck A, *et al.* Hopelessness and eventual suicide: a ten-year prospective study of patients hospitalised with suicidal ideation. *Am J Psychiatry.* 1985; **142**: 559–63.

37 Rigby S, *et al.* Quality of life assessment in MND: development of the Social Withdrawal Scale. *J Neurol Sci.* 2002; **169**: 26–34.

38 Young J, McNicholl P. Against all odds: positive life experience of people with advanced amyotrophic lateral sclerosis. *Health Soc Work.* 1998; **23**: 35–43.

39 Brown J, Addington-Hall J. How people with motor neurone disease talk about living with their illness: a narrative study. *J Adv Nurs.* 2008; 62(2): 200–8.

40 Ray RA, Street AF. Caregiver bodywork: family members' experiences of caring for a person with motor neurone disease. *J Adv Nurs.* 2006; 56(1): 35–43.

41 Paz S, Seymour JE. Pain: theories, evaluation, management. In: Payne S, Seymour JE, Ingleton C, editors. *Palliative Care Nursing: principles and evidence for practice.* Buckingham: Open University Press; 2008. pp. 252–89.

42 McCaffery M. *Nursing Practice Theories Related to Cognition, Bodily Pain, and Man-Environmental Interaction.* Los Angeles: UCLA Students Store; 1968.

43 Fink R, Gates R. Pain assessment. In: Ferrell B, Coyle N, editors. *Textbook of Palliative Nursing.* New York: Oxford University Press; 2001. pp. 53–71.

44 Twycross R, Wilcock A. *Symptom Management in Advanced Cancer.* 3rd ed. Oxford: Radcliffe Medical Press; 2002.

45 Ashburn MA, Staats PS. Management of chronic pain. *Lancet.* 1999; 353(9167): 1865–9.

46 World Health Organization. WHO's pain ladder. Available at: www.who.int/cancer/palliative/painladder/en/ (accessed 5 February 2009).

47 Sykes N. End of life care. In: Oliver D, Borasio GD, Walsh D, editors. *Palliative Care in Amyotrophic Lateral Sclerosis.* Oxford: Oxford University Press; 2006. pp. 287–300.

48 Henry C, Seymour JE. *Advance Care Planning: a guide for health and social care professionals.* Leicester: NHS End of Life Care Programme; 2007.

49 National Council for Palliative Care. *Changing Gear: guidelines for managing the last days of life in adults.* London: NCPC; 2006.

50 National Institute for Health and Clinical Excellence. *Guidance on Cancer Services: improving supportive and palliative care for adults with cancer.* London: NICE; 2004.

CHAPTER 4

Symptom relief in palliative neurological care

Annette Edwards

Many symptoms are shared across neurological conditions and can significantly affect a patient's quality of life. Good symptom control depends on thorough history taking, careful examination and relevant investigations, enabling the professional to draw an overall picture of the likely disease process and how it is affecting the individual and their carers. Open discussion with the patient (and carers where appropriate) is important and therapeutic, involving explanation of the likely cause of the problem and discussing options regarding management, including the advantages and disadvantages of treatments. While many supportive interventions have not been the subject of robust clinical trials, there is accepted best clinical practice,[1] and the patient should be reassured that the whole team will work together to try and control symptoms and maximise their quality of life. This chapter reviews a range of common problems and their management, drawing on the author's clinical practice and available published evidence.

DIFFICULTY WALKING

This can be due to a variety of causes and needs to be fully assessed and managed appropriately. The following should be considered.
➤ Leg weakness may be distal or proximal.
➤ Spasticity causes a stiffness and jerkiness of gait and toe catching.
➤ Patients with Parkinson's disease (PD) typically walk in a stooped position with a slow shuffling gait and narrow base, and have a tendency to fall.
➤ Ataxia, with a broad based unstable gait, can be due to cerebellar causes, often associated with nystagmus and dysarthria, or sensory loss due to a

peripheral sensory lesion, e.g. polyneuropathy. If the latter, it tends to be worse if there is loss of other sensory input, e.g. in the dark.

➤ Frontal lobe disease can cause apraxia, with disturbed central organisation of walking, and is often associated with incontinence or dementia.

➤ Pain from a variety of causes can interfere with mobility.

Management is aimed at ensuring safety and helping to maintain a patient's independence where possible. Thorough assessment by a physiotherapist is vital.

WEAKNESS

Weakness is a common symptom of advanced neurological disease. In the lower limbs it may present as foot drop, a tendency to trip, difficulty rising from chairs and excessive fatigue on walking. It can be equally disabling in the upper limbs, causing flail arms if proximal muscles are involved or, with distal muscle weakness, difficulty with fine movements, e.g. opening bottles and turning keys, and a tendency to drop things.

The introduction of aids and appliances because of increasing weakness needs to be handled sensitively. Patients may see this as further evidence of deterioration; however, appropriate aids should significantly improve a patient's quality of life. Appropriate equipment needs to be accessed in a timely manner, with the patient's situation under constant review. Needs vary and may be addressed by simple interventions such as splints, light weight cutlery and wheelchairs. However, adjustments to the home may be required, such as walk-in showers or environmental control systems.

PAIN

With the exception of multiple sclerosis (MS), pain is often not recognised as a major problem in many patients with long-term neurological conditions. However, it is frequently overlooked, unless asked for directly. There are several possible aetiological factors, and patients may have more than one pain syndrome. In MS, acute or chronic pain syndromes occur in 30–80% of patients[2] and pain has been reported in up to 73% patients with motor neurone disease (MND).[3]

Musculo-skeletal pain

Restricted movement may result in stiff joints and potentially painful contractures. In addition, reduced muscle tone around joints will affect positioning and may result in joint dislocation, commonly of the shoulders. Physiotherapy has an important role to play, assessing positioning, ensuring adequate and effective support, teaching passive movements to help prevent contractures and encouraging active exercise where appropriate. Pharmacological and other non pharmacological approaches may also be of benefit.

➤ The application of heat and transcutaneous electrical nerve stimulation (TENS).

➤ Paracetamol and non steroidal anti inflammatory drugs (NSAIDs) are often helpful.

➤ NSAID gel applied to a localised area may be helpful.

➤ Opioids may be occasionally needed if the pain is severe and doesn't respond to the above.[4] Weak opioids may be sufficient, e.g. codeine in combination with paracetamol, but if pain is still a problem despite, e.g. co-codamol 30/500 qds, then a stronger opioid should be prescribed. A short acting opioid, e.g. morphine liquid, is useful for dose titration and may also be used half an hour prior to anticipated painful events. If pain is a persistent problem then regular slow release opioids may be required. Transdermal opioids, e.g buprenorphine or fentanyl patches, can be particularly useful if the patient has difficulty swallowing

Skin pressure

As patients become more debilitated their mobility is reduced, and they spend longer in a chair or bed, often unable to change position themselves. Attention to pressure area care is very important. Pressure sores are a major cause of pain and distress, and patients may need analgesics, working up the World Health Organization (WHO) analgesic ladder as required (*see* Chapter 3). Attention to dressings and positioning are vital. In established pressure sores, topical opioids may be useful.[5]

Neuropathic pain

This is particularly problematic in MS, including painful paroxysmal symptoms and burning dysaesthesias. Central pain from sclerotic plaque lesions affecting pain pathways in the central nervous system is reported in around 33% of patients with MS.[6]

The following medications have been shown to be useful in neuropathic pain.

➤ Tricyclic antidepressants.[7] Pain may be controlled on a lower dose than traditionally used as an antidepressant, e.g. amitriptyline 10–50 mg nocte. Side effects include dry mouth and sedation, which may be advantageous.

➤ Antiepileptics. Traditionally carbamazepine has been used for trigeminal neuralgia. More recently gabapentin and pregabalin[8,9] have been used for neuropathic pain. These are normally well tolerated and have the advantage of few drug interactions.

➤ Opioids have been shown to be effective for neuropathic pain,[10,11] and may need to be considered if the above measures are not helpful.

➤ The role of cannabinoids, e.g. oral dronabinol in pain control is still uncertain, although studies suggest some benefit in central pain.[12,13] Some patients, particularly those with MS, use cannabis, claiming it helps relieve pain and spasm. However, owing to the legal status of the drug, it has implications for healthcare workers involved, who cannot endorse its use.

Muscle spasm and cramps

Combined non pharmacological and pharmacological approaches may be necessary.

➤ Multi-professional assessment and management of spasticity is essential (*see* below).

➤ Painful cramps may respond to stretching and physiotherapy.

➤ Some patients report benefit from quinine 200–300 mg nocte.

➤ Systematic reviews have shown some evidence that antispasmodics/muscle relaxants may be helpful, although it is unclear as to their comparative efficacy and safety.[14,15,16] Alternatives include:
  - baclofen 5–20 mg tid
  - tizanidine 2–24 mg daily in 3–4 divided doses
  - diazepam 5 mg nocte increasing to 10 mg qds
  - clonazepam 1–4 mg nocte
  - dantrolene 25–100 mg qds.

  Their use is restricted by unwanted side effects, e.g. muscle weakness (possibly greater with baclofen and dantrolene), drowsiness and dry mouth (tizanidine). Dantrolene acts peripherally on the muscle contractile system, and hence causes muscle weakness. There are also reports of hepatotoxicity.

➤ Painful tonic spasms may also respond to antiepileptics, e.g. gabapentin, carbamazepine.

➤ TENS may be useful in treating pain and muscle spasm.[17]

SPASTICITY

Spasticity is a common symptom in MS, affecting between 40 and 60% of all patients, but is also seen in other advanced neurological diseases with upper motor neurone damage. It can cause pain, stiffness and muscle spasm, resulting in significant immobility and restricted activities of daily living, for example affecting a person's ability to walk, transfer, wash and dress themselves. Spasticity may vary day to day, and may be exacerbated by a noxious stimulus, e.g. pressure sores, constipation. Untreated spasticity can lead to the development of contractures, which may further exacerbate pain and problems with hygiene and activities, as well as predisposing to ulceration.

A team approach is essential, addressing issues such as fatigue management, provision of specialised equipment and psychological support, e.g. with regard to altered body image, sexuality and role changes. Physiotherapists may help with positioning, active and passive exercise, and the assessment of mobility. In addition, care should be aimed at preventing the development of pressure sores, urinary infections and constipation. Pharmacotherapy has a role in spasticity, but needs to be considered carefully; the following approaches may warrant exploration.

➤ Antispasmodic medication may be useful (*see* above) However, it may unmask weakness and fatigue in the muscles involved, and potentially transfers and mobility may deteriorate.

➤ Intrathecal baclofen is theoretically a useful alternative for diffuse severe spasticity as it can bypass the blood brain barrier, concentrating mainly at the level of the motor neurones with little cerebral diffusion. Following a successful bolus intrathecal test an intrathecal administration device is implanted. The daily dose can be reset as required until a constant baseline effect is achieved.[18] Continuous intrathecal baclofen infusions have been shown to improve function and quality of life[19,20] with reduction of spasticity and spasms.

➤ Botulinum toxin injections are effective in reducing focal spasticity and are associated with functional benefit.[15] If useful they can be repeated at 3–4 month intervals.

➤ Occasionally peripheral neurotomies may be indicated for focal spasticity or dystonia.

➤ Cannabinoids may be effective in reducing muscle spasticity and pain through their action on cannabinoid receptors (CB1) in the CNS. Studies in patients with MS suggest benefit in both spasticity and related pain.[13,21,22] However, it is still questionable whether cannabinoids are superior to existing conventional medications for the treatment of pain and spasticity.[23] In addition, adverse effects, e.g. dizziness can be quite significant.

MOVEMENT DISORDERS

These occur predominantly in PD and Huntington's disease (HD) and fall into two groups.

1 Reduction in movement (bradykinesia, akinesia).

2 Hyperkinetic involuntary movements, e.g. tremor, dystonia, chorea, myoclonus, tics. These are examined below.

Tremor

➤ Rest tremor is a cardinal symptom of PD and may improve with high dose dopaminergic medication.

➤ Anticholinergics, e.g. benzhexol may also be useful but can cause confusion.

➤ Botulinum toxin injections into forearm muscles (predominantly flexors) may be effective.[24,25,26] Adverse effects include focal weakness of extensor muscles, interfering with fine motor movements of hands. The procedure takes approximately 1 week for a response and lasts 3–4 months.

➤ Botulinum injections for jaw tremor have also been described.[27]

➤ Rarely surgical intervention is considered for severe tremor or dystonia, including thalamotomy, pallidotomy and deep brain stimulation.

Dystonia

➤ Sustained muscle contractions cause twisting and repetitive movements or abnormal postures, and may be localised or generalised.

➤ Levodopa may improve or exacerbate dystonia.

➤ Results following treatment with botulinum toxin injections have been variable,[28] although it may be helpful for painful foot dystonia.[29]

➤ Botulinum A and botulinum B injections are proven to be effective interventions in cervical dystonia.[30,31,32]

Blepharospasm is a form of focal dystonia, with initially uncontrollable blinking and then involuntary, forcible closure of the eyelids. It can be problematic in patients with progressive supranuclear palsy (PSP) and PD. Botulinum toxin injections into the orbicularis oculi muscles may be functionally beneficial, sometimes with the addition of anticholinergic drugs and possibly lid crutches.

Chorea

➤ Jerky quasi-purposeful movements seen especially in HD.

➤ Neuroleptics may help both chorea and the psychiatric symptoms of HD, e.g. haloperidol, fluphenazine.[33]

➤ Atypical neuroleptics have a reduced risk of extrapyramidal side effects but may cause more weight gain, e.g. clozapine, olanzapine.[34]

➤ Tetrabenazine, which depletes dopamine from nerve terminals, has been shown to reduce chorea severity but not gait or parkinsonism.[35]

RESPIRATORY PROBLEMS

Breathlessness

Breathlessness in patients with progressive neurological disease can have several causes.

1 Lower respiratory infection. This may be due to respiratory muscle weakness with poor chest expansion, difficulty producing an effective cough to clear secretions, and compounding aspiration.
2 Pulmonary emboli, associated with reduced mobility.
3 Weakness of muscles of respiration – particularly in MND, which may be aggravated by poor nutrition. Both the diaphragm and intercostal muscles may be involved.
4 Co-existent cardiac or lung pathology.

Management will depend on the cause. If this is thought to be due to an infection then appropriate antibiotics and physiotherapy may be useful. Vaccination against influenza virus should be considered in patients with advanced neurological disease. If aspiration is a contributing factor then alternative methods of feeding need to be considered and discussed. Non invasive ventilation provides good symptom relief for symptoms due to hypoventilation and hypoxia (*see* below). The following symptomatic approaches may be beneficial.

➤ Positioning – sitting upright and supported.
➤ A flow of air over the face, e.g. a fan or open window.
➤ Breathing exercises, relaxation and reassurance.
➤ A recent Cochrane review[36] concluded that walking aids, neuro-electrical muscle stimulation, and chest wall vibration appear to be effective in a variety of patients with advanced disease, although most studies have been done in patients with chronic obstructive pulmonary disease.

PHARMACOLOGICAL TREATMENTS

➤ Opioids are effective in relieving breathlessness,[4,37] e.g. oral morphine, initially 2–5 mg 4 hourly and titrating as required.
➤ Benzodiazepines will help with associated anxiety and panic, e.g. diazepam 2–5 mg nocte/tid, or lorazepam 0.5–1 mg[38,39] which may be given sublingually in an acute attack. However, these drugs need to be given in small doses and titrated carefully in light of the patient's poor respiratory reserve.
➤ Selective serotonin reuptake inhibitors (SSRIs) are safe and useful for panic and anxiety as a longer-term measure.

Ventilatory insufficiency

In patients with MND, weakness of respiratory muscles develops as the disease progresses. Some patients present with respiratory insufficiency.[40] While patients are not normally symptomatic until their forced expiratory volume (FEV) falls below 50% predicted, it is variable, and some may develop respiratory failure (defined as arterial or ear lobe $pCO_2 > 6.5\,kPa$) with a vital capacity (VC) as high as 75%.[41] This may occur in the absence of breathlessness at rest or orthopnoea. VC is not always a good measure of respiratory function, particularly in patients with bulbar symptoms, and other measures are used, e.g. sniff nasal pressure.[41,42]

One of the earliest indications of respiratory insufficiency in MND is sleep disturbance. Hypoventilation initially occurs in REM sleep when accessory muscles are less active, and ventilation becomes more dependent on the diaphragm, which functions less efficiently in the supine position. During the night episodes of hypoventilation and associated oxygen desaturation may cause recurrent arousal. The development of nocturnal hypercapnia may then contribute to impaired concentration, drowsiness, morning headache, nausea, irritability, anorexia and depression. Dyspnoea on exertion or talking may be present. If hypoxia is suspected, following discussion with the patient, a referral should be made to a respiratory physician for a full respiratory assessment. Overnight arterial oxygen saturation measurement can be obtained at home by means of a small device that attaches to a finger. The results can then be communicated to the respiratory team in the morning.

Symptoms due to hypoventilation may be dramatically improved with non invasive positive pressure ventilation (NIPPV). These masked ventilatory systems include devices that deliver intermittent inspiratory positive pressure (e.g. 'NIPPY', B & D Electromedical, UK) or bi-level positive pressure devices which deliver different levels of positive pressure in inspiration and expiration (BiPAP). There are many different interfaces available, including nasal mask, full face mask and nasal cushions, but soreness or ulceration of the nose can be problematic. Small portable machines are available. Using NIPPV requires reasonable dexterity, and patients may be unable to manage it themselves, placing an extra burden on carers. Patients with pronounced bulbar symptoms may have difficulties with NIPPV, with episodes of obstruction related to abnormal function of the vocal cords, and increased risk of aspiration.[42]

When respiratory problems are anticipated, for example in patients with MND, it is important to start discussions early, to give patients time to ask questions and begin to consider if respiratory support is something they might wish for themselves. A randomised controlled trial found a medium survival benefit of about seven months in patients with good bulbar function using non invasive ventilation, accompanied by improvement in quality of life measures.[43] Once established, patients often start using non invasive ventilation during the night, but as the disease progresses they may find it beneficial to use for periods during the day. Increasing dependency on the ventilator is likely and the limits of treatment need to be explained.

Invasive ventilation via tracheostomy protects the airway from secretions and can prolong life as the disease progresses. It is rarely carried out in the UK and raises complex ethical issues. When a patient with MND is ventilated acutely, with or without an established diagnosis, independence from the ventilator is rarely achieved.[44] Hence, it is essential that ventilation and end of life care issues should be discussed with the patient and carers long before an emergency arises, and decisions carefully documented.

Cough

Cough is often weak and ineffectual, and may be triggered by attempts at swallowing. Coughing and choking episodes are common in patients with MND but infrequently associated with overt chest infection.[45] Treatment should be of the underlying cause. Opioids may be helpful if cough remains troublesome.[4]

Clinical management would include the following.

➤ Identifying and treating infection as appropriate.
➤ Considering physiotherapy; patients and carers can be taught techniques to assist expiratory movement during cough.
➤ Portable home suction devices to remove secretions.
➤ A mechanical insufflation-exsufflation device ('cough assist') increases expiratory flow rates and may help clear secretions and mucus plugging.
➤ If there are concerns about aspiration consider alternative ways of feeding.
➤ Cough can be precipitated by acid reflux – consider for example metoclopramide, use of proton pump inhibitors.
➤ If there is difficult expectoration thick secretions consider:
  • nebulised saline to loosen secretions, or humidifier;
  • carbocisteine 250–750 mg tid.
➤ Occasionally nebulised local anaesthetic for nocturnal cough is useful.

Choking (laryngospasm)/respiratory distress

Episodes of laryngospasm, paroxysms of coughing and inspiratory stridor with concomitant apnoea, usually only last a few seconds, but can be very frightening. They can occur during the day or night, and may be triggered by gastro-oesphageal reflux, or by inhalation of noxious chemicals or smoke.[46] Episodes may be prevented by giving antisecretory and prokinetic drugs before each meal, and avoiding eating before going to sleep. In an acute situation, sitting up, fixing the arms to stabilise the body, and slowing breathing may be beneficial. If the respiratory distress continues, sublingual lorazepam may help.

SWALLOWING PROBLEMS

Approximately 80% patients with MND will eventually develop significant bulbar problems, but difficulties with swallowing are also present in the later stages of MS, PD and HD. Chewing and swallowing becomes difficult and tiring, with frequent choking, regurgitation and food sticking. Around 21% patients with MND are malnourished.[47] In some this is due to dysphagia, but drooling and slow speed completing meals causes social embarrassment. Arm weakness also slows eating and renders patients dependent on others for adequate food and liquid intake.

Management includes the following.[42]

➤ Involvement of a speech and language therapist (SALT) to assess the cause of swallowing problems, advise on safe swallowing techniques, and contribute to decisions on gastrostomy placement, working in close collaboration with the dietician.

➤ Modifying the texture and consistency of food (blending food, thickening drinks).

➤ Advising on changes in posture and head position may be useful, e.g. eating upright with chin tucked in, which will help to protect the airway.

➤ Consideration of alternative feeding methods.

Gastrostomy feeding should be considered to limit weight loss, or to ease distressing coughing and choking episodes at meal times and risk of aspiration. Discussions about this should take place early in the disease process. There is a higher risk when procedures are carried out when the patient already has developed poor respiratory reserve. The risk of death in the month following PEG insertion is small if the lung vital capacity (VC) is greater than 50%.[48] Gastrostomy tubes can be placed either with the support of endoscopy (PEGs) or under radiological control (RIGs).[42] Radiological insertion of gastrostomy is often better tolerated, as little or no sedation is required and hence it can be considered in patients with compromised respiratory function. PEG feeding has been shown to decrease weight loss and improve survival and quality of life in patients with MND.[48]

SIALORRHOEA/DROOLING

Sialorrhoea (excessive drooling of saliva) is a common symptom in a number of PLTNCs, especially PD (70–80%) and MND (20–30%). Saliva production is mediated by submandibular, sublingual and parotid glands, which are innervated by the parasympathetic nervous system. The submandibular and sublingual glands are responsible for the majority of the baseline, more viscous saliva. The parotid glands produce thin serous secretions, particularly during eating and drinking. Stimulation of the muscarinic receptor M3 by the neurotransmitter acetylcholine is thought to induce salivation. However, the flow of saliva can also be enhanced by sympathetic innervations, which increase contraction of muscle fibres around salivary ducts.

Sialorrhoea is mainly due to infrequent and difficult swallowing, with poor facial and oral neuromuscular control. Patients may have difficulty manipulating saliva in the mouth. The situation is complicated in PD as it may be exacerbated by a tendency to keep the mouth open and a stooped posture. In general salivary production is actually reduced in PD.[49] However, occasionally there is evidence of autonomic dysfunction causing oesophageal dysphagia and hypersecretion of saliva. In addition, excess secretions can be stimulated by inflammation (e.g. dental caries and gingivitis, gastro-oesophageal reflux) and certain medications (e.g. clozapine). Drooling has a significant effect on a patient's quality of life, causing skin irritation, infections, foul mouth odour, aspiration, embarrassment and increased dependency.[50]

Non pharmacological approaches

The following approaches may be useful either alone or in combination with medications.

➤ SALT interventions including patient education regarding drooling and swallowing, instruction to consciously swallow more often, and use of a brooch-style device that emits a beep at regular intervals reminding patients to swallow have been shown to be effective in mild disease.[51]

➤ Training patients to stabilise head position; provision of a head-back wheelchair.

➤ Home suction device.

Pharmacological approaches

The following medications are used in clinical practice.

a. Anticholinergics

Use of these is limited by side effects of constipation, confusion, dry mouth, urinary retention, blurred vision and dizziness. They are contra-indicated in patients with cardiac arrhythmias, closed angle glaucoma and prostatic hypertrophy. Most studies have been carried out in children with, for example, cerebral palsy.[52]

Options would be:

i Hyoscine hydrobromide patches, 1 mg over 72 hours, 1–3 patches titrated according to response. Studies have confirmed their benefit in children with drooling.[53,54] Local irritation and pruritis at patch site can be a problem.

ii Atropine. Open label studies in patients with bulbar MND[55] or PD and

PSP[56] have shown reductions in objective and subjective measures of saliva production after 1 week. The usual preparation (although unlicensed) is atropine eyedrops 0.5%, 2 drops (0.5 mg) bd–qds sublingually. It is also available in tablet or liquid form, 300–600 mcg bd–tid.

  iii Glycopyrrolate. This does not cross the blood brain barrier and hence should have fewer central effects. It is the most evaluated of the anticholinergic agents to date,[57,58,59] although there is only one randomised, double-blind, placebo controlled study,[60] in which there was a significant improvement in subjective drooling score, but a 30% dropout rate. It can be used in the following preparations:
- subcutaneous infusion, 1.2 mg over 24 hours[3]
- tablets, 1 or 2 mg. 0.5 mg od–tid titrated to maximum of 8 mg/day in adults
- nebulised glycopyrrolate.[61]

  iv Other anticholinergic drugs that may be useful include:
- benztropine[62]
- benzhexol[63]
- ipratropium bromide spray sublingual.[64]

  v Amitriptyline. Low doses, e.g. 10–25 mg nocte, can help dry secretions and improve sleep and anxiety.

b. Beta blockers
If anticholinergic drugs are not helpful, or if the secretions are very viscous, a trial of for example propanolol 10 mg tid can be considered, but it can exacerbate fatigue.[65]

Botulinum toxin

This neurotoxin produced by clostridium botulinum blocks acetylcholine release from cholinergic neurosecretory junctions and hence prevents stimulation of the salivary gland. Injections are carried out into parotid and/or submandibular glands. Most research has been done into this, with encouraging open label studies and randomised controlled trials.

Four randomised controlled trials have investigated botulinum toxin type A in patients with PD, MND, multiple system atrophy (MSA) and corticobasal degeneration. These have demonstrated statistically significant reductions in saliva production according to both objective[66,67,68] and subjective analysis.[66,67,69] Measures of familial and social distress and embarrassment are also improved.[67]

One random controlled trial of botulinum toxin type B in sialorrhoea showed no statistically significant decrease in objective measures but statistically significant improvements in various subjective scales.[70] However, the benefit may vary in different patient groups: in an open label study of botulinum toxin B,[71] patients with MS had a shorter benefit duration and higher prevalence of viscous saliva compared with those with PD.

Botulinum toxin injections are generally well tolerated, with more than 80% of patients satisfied with treatment and willing to receive repeat injections.[67,71] Any adverse effects are usually mild, comprising of dry mouth, transient flu-like symptoms, injection site discomfort and thickened saliva. However, there is a risk of transitory difficulty in swallowing. They have been shown to be as efficient as scopolamine, but with fewer adverse effects.[72] There is still some uncertainty about the optimum dose, with botulinum A 75 MU injected into each parotid gland being more effective than lower doses.[68] In addition, there is debate as to the necessity of ultrasound guided treatment,[66] although it is probably more important when injecting submandibular glands, as these are in a less accessible location. The beneficial effects usually last between 3 and 8 months, and can be repeated.

Radiotherapy

Radiation of the parotid gland is often effective,[73,74] although the dose required to produce salivary gland atrophy varies between patients. Typically a patient will be offered radiotherapy to one side first, with the option of radiotherapy to another gland if there has been no significant benefit. Adverse effects include skin soreness, which may take a few weeks to settle. Xerostomia may last months or years.[75] There is an increased risk of late malignancy in the irradiated field 10–15 years post treatment, although this is not of particular concern in patients with short prognosis. There is also a risk of osteonecrosis of the jaw.

Surgery

In severe sialorrhoea that is unresponsive to pharmacotherapy or radiotherapy, surgery may be considered. Procedures include the following.[76]

➤ Transtympanic neurectomy. This relatively simple surgery is performed through the middle ear and does not require a general anaesthetic, but it can affect taste. The nerve fibres often regenerate within 6–18 months.

➤ Submandibular or parotid gland excision.

➤ Submandibular or parotid duct relocation.

A typical procedure is a combination of parotid duct ligation with submandibular gland excision or duct rerouting. However, this is a significant operation resulting in severe irreversible xerostomia, and a risk of sialocele and dental caries. In addition, there is an external scar and potentially facial weakness after submandibular excision.

SPEECH

Many patients may develop difficulties with vocalisation, ranging from quiet speech to dysarthria and anarthria. Slurring of speech, caused by impaired tongue movements, usually presents before dysphagia. Management includes advice on strategies to optimise the intelligibility of speech, and voice amplification may be useful for patients with good articulation but a weak voice due to respiratory muscle weakness. Alternatives to speech will need to be considered as the disease progresses, including writing, communication devices (e.g. 'Lightwriter®'), switches and scanning systems, alphabet boards and individualised communication charts. While a partner or carer may still understand the patient's speech, early introduction to the speech and language therapist to develop alternative means of communication is important to aid wider communication.

CONSTIPATION

This is a common symptom in advanced neurological disease, and has many causes. Weakness, including reduced power of the abdominal muscles to push, loss of mobility, effects of medications, especially anticholinergics, a low residue diet and dehydration, may all contribute. It may also be a sign of autonomic dysfunction, with delayed gastric emptying of solids and impaired colonic motility after eating.[77] Prevention of constipation is important, by ensuring adequate hydration, a balanced diet and aperients.

Management may involve the following.

➤ Where possible the cause should be addressed, e.g. stopping medications, dietary advice.
➤ Ensuring adequate hydration.
➤ Laxatives – a combination of stimulant and softener is useful, e.g.:
  • co-danthramer or condanthrusate (5–10 mL bd, titrating as required);
  • senna and lactulose (5–10 mL bd);
  • movicol (1–2 sachets od, increasing up to a maximum of 8 per day).
➤ Faecal incontinence may be related to loss of normal sensation, but management should exclude impaction and overflow.
➤ Consider referral to the district nursing service.

URINARY DIFFICULTIES

These affect 50–75% MS patients, but are also common in PD. Late stage HD patients may lose bowel and bladder control.[78] Bladder symptoms can result in social isolation, difficulties with sexual activity and decreased self esteem, as well as creating secondary health problems, such as urinary tract infections. The most common is urgency, often with associated urinary frequency and urge incontinence.[79] The severity of symptoms relates to the degree of pyramidal impairment in the lower limbs, reflecting the extent of spinal involvement. The following medications may be useful:

➤ anticholinergic or smooth muscles relaxants, e.g. propantheline, oxybutynin
➤ anticholinergic antidepressants can also be useful – imipramine, amitriptyline
➤ intranasal desmopressin can be effective for increased voiding frequency and incontinence, and is well tolerated.[80]

In addition, patients may benefit from referral to the district nursing service or a specialist continence service for assessment and advice. Pads or a convene sheath should be offered.

Urinary hesitancy or retention may be due to poor or absent detrusor contractions. Occasionally bethanechol is useful, but often catheterisation is needed. If patients are still reasonably mobile and independent, intermittent self catheterisation may be preferable, reducing the likelihood of urinary tract infections while relieving symptoms.

COGNITIVE AND MOOD RELATED PROBLEMS
Anxiety

Anxiety affects many patients, and can be particularly troublesome at night. Reassurance, practical support and attention to symptom control are important. Patients may benefit from formal psychological support, such as cognitive or behavioural techniques, or from pharmacological interventions. Short acting benzodiazepines, e.g. temazepam 10–20 mg nocte will help with anxiety precluding sleep. Panic attacks during the day may be helped by lorazepam 0.5–1 mg which may be used sublingually. If anxiety persists throughout the day a longer acting benzodiazepine, e.g. diazepam 5 mg nocte is preferable, or SSRIs. Citalopram has the advantage of being available in drop formulation, so the dose can be titrated slowly.

Depression

Sadness, depression and grief are frequent features in patients with a PLTNC,[78,81,82,83] exacerbated by the uncertainty of prognosis, increasing dependency and often loss of role in the family. This may lead to an all pervading sense of hopelessness and loss of self worth. Patients and carers should be offered both practical and psychological support. Conventional antidepressants, e.g. SSRIs may need to be considered.[81] Amitriptyline and mirtazepine may also be useful.[33]

Dementia

This is common in late stage PD and HD, and can put significant strain on carers. In addition, about 50% of people with MS have a degree of cognitive impairment.[84] Frontotemporal dementia occurs in approx 5% patients with MND.[42] Patients may initially display disinhibited behaviour and difficulties in planning complex tasks and decision making. As it progresses they may display rigid behaviour and become withdrawn. A higher proportion have more subtle cognitive involvement (20–40%), which appears to be more common in patients with predominantly bulbar symptoms rather than limb involvement.[85]

Frank psychosis in patients with advanced neurological disease is rare but does occur in HD. It may be helped by antipsychotics such as resperidone[33]. Olanzapine, haloperidol, and buspirone may be useful for behavioural symptoms of HD.[33]

Emotional lability

This is a recognised feature of patients with PLTNCs, especially MS.[86] In addition, some patients have spontaneous, pathological episodes of laughing and crying (pseudobulbar effect), despite an underlying affective tone that is normal, which can be very distressing. This occurs in approx 10% of MS patients[87] and up to 50% of patients with MND.[88]

Patients may be helped by the following:

➤ SSRIs – these may be beneficial at a lower dose than needed for depression[89]

➤ amitriptyline or similar tricyclic antidepressant

➤ there is also some evidence for the use of dextromethorphan and quinidine.[90]

SLEEP DISORDERS

Sleep disturbances in patients with advanced neurological disease are common, often severe, and are typically under recognised and ineffectively treated. Insomnia may be due to pain, anxiety, depression, cough due to excess secretions, and hypoxia causing frequent nocturnal wakening and daytime drowsiness. Excessive daytime sleepiness can be a problem, particularly with PD and MS, where it may be due to the disease, or medications. The stimulant, modafinil, 200 mg od, may be useful.[91,92]

FATIGUE

Fatigue is a frequent debilitating symptom in patients with PLTNCs.[93] Potential contributing factors include a poor sleeping pattern, nocturia, chronic pain, medication (e.g. antispasticity and antidepressant drugs), depression and negative coping strategies. A thorough holistic assessment is essential, and education on energy conservation and the provision of suitable aids and equipment may be useful.

SEXUAL DYSFUNCTION

Patients may not readily disclose sexual problems, despite them causing significant distress, but may respond to sensitive questioning around how the illness is affecting their relationships. Physical factors contributing to sexual dysfunction include weakened pelvic muscles, spasticity, general fatigue, disturbances in the autonomic nervous system and the effects of medications. In addition, psychological factors related to depression and anxiety, altered body image and change in role within a relationship are equally important.[94]

Management may involve the following:[95]

➤ explanation, psychological support and counselling, which may require referral to specialist services

➤ optimal management of physical symptoms, including pain and spasticity

➤ rationalising medications, e.g. antidepressants, beta blockers

➤ use of sildenafil or intracavernous papaverine.

OTHER NEUROLOGICAL SYMPTOMS

Patients with advanced neurological disease may have many symptoms related to their disease. These include unsteadiness, feeling light headed, altered consciousness, visual disturbance, such as optic neuropathy in MS, vertigo, tinnitus and epilepsy. These need to be fully assessed and managed appropriately. Reduced sensation increases the risk of developing skin ulcers and infection, and good skincare and education is essential.

Autonomic dysfunction is increasingly being recognised as a feature of many neurological conditions, including MSA, PD, MS and MND. Sweating disturbances are common and distressing symptoms of PD that are related mainly to autonomic dysfunction, off periods, and dyskinesias.[96] Axial hyperhidrosis may be a compensatory phenomenon for reduced sympathetic function in the extremities, with decreased palmar sweating.[97] Autonomic dysfunction has also been reported in severely affected MND patients.[98,99]

CONCLUSION

Ongoing thorough assessment and optimal management of symptoms is important for patients with progressive neurological disease. Symptoms vary greatly; not only between different conditions, but also within each disease, and in terms of those experienced by each person over time. This makes long-term planning difficult. Studies have shown the value of key worker roles and a multidisciplinary approach, and also the importance of user involvement and self managed care.[100]

Close liaison with the primary care team is essential, with the general practitioner (GP) involved from the outset. In the UK National Health Service, day to day management of symptoms depends on the GP. Even though progressive long-term neurological conditions are relatively rare, GPs are familiar with palliative and end of life care in cancer, and similar principles apply. Also, referrals to community services and local palliative care teams are often initiated by the GP.

With careful attention to detail, quality of life can be good, even when the disease is advanced. The challenge is to match care with the ever changing needs of the individual and their family.

REFERENCES

1 Andersen PM, Borasio GD, Dengler R, *et al.* EFNS task force on management of amyotrophic lateral sclerosis: guidelines for diagnosing and clinical care of patients and relatives. *Eur J Neurol.* 2005; **12**: 921–38.

2 Solaro C, Tanganelli P, Messmer UM. Pharmacological treatment of pain in multiple sclerosis. *Expert Rev Neurother.* 2007; **7**(9): 1165–74, 87.

3 Oliver D. The quality of care and symptom control – the effects on the terminal phase of MND/ALS. *J Neurol Sci.* 1996; **139**(Suppl.): S134–6.

4 Oliver D. Opioid medication in the palliative care of motor neurone disease. *Palliat Med.* 1998; **12**: 113–15.

5 Flock P. Pilot study to determine the effectiveness of diamorphine gel to control pressure ulcer pain. *J Pain Symptom Manage.* 2003; **25**(6): 547–4.

6 Boivie J. Central pain. In: Wall PD, Melzack R, editors. *Textbook of Pain.* New York: Churchill Livingstone; 1999. pp. 879–914.

7 Saarto T, Wiffen PJ. Antidepressants for neuropathic pain. *Cochrane Database Syst Rev.* 2007; **4**: CD005454.

8 Gray P. Pregabalin in the management of central neuropathic pain. *Expert Opin Pharmacother.* 2007; **8**(17): 3035–41.

9 Finnerup NB, Jensen TS. Clinical use of pregabalin in the management of central neuropathic pain. *Neuropsychiatr Dis Treat.* 2007; **3**(6): 885–91.

10 Eisenberg E, McNicol ED, Carr DB. Efficacy and safety of opioid agonists in the treatment of neuropathic pain of nonmalignant origin: systematic review and meta-analysis of randomized controlled trials. *JAMA.* 2005; **293**(24): 3043–52.

11 Eisenberg E, McNicol ED, Carr DB. Opioids for neuropathic pain. *Cochrane Database Syst Rev.* 2006; **3**: CD006146.

12 Svendsen KB, Jensen TS, Bach FW. Does the cannabinoid dronabinol reduce central pain in multiple sclerosis? Randomised double blind placebo controlled crossover trial. *BMJ.* 2004; **329**(7460): 253.

13 Barnes MP. Sativex®: clinical efficacy and tolerability in the treatment of symptoms of multiple sclerosis and neuropathic pain. *Expert Opin Pharmacother.* 2006; **7**(5): 607–15.

14 Chou R, Peterson K, Helfand M. Comparative efficacy and safety of skeletal muscle relaxants for spasticity and musculoskeletal conditions: a systematic review. *J Pain Symptom Manage.* 2004; **28**(2): 140–75.

15 Beard S, Hunn A, Wight J. Treatments for spasticity and pain in multiple sclerosis: a systematic review. *Health Technol Assess.* 2003; **7**(40): iii, ix–x, 1–111.

16 Paisley S, Beard S, Hunn A, *et al.* Clinical effectiveness of oral treatments for spasticity in multiple sclerosis: a systematic review. *Mult Scler.* 2002; **8**(4): 319–29.

17 Miller L, Mattison P, Paul L, *et al.* The effects of transcutaneous electrical nerve stimulation (TENS) on spasticity in multiple sclerosis. *Mult Scler.* 2007; **13**(4): 527–33.

18 Dones I, Nazzi G, Broggi G. The guidelines for the diagnosis and treatment of spasticity. *J Neurosurg Sci.* 2006; **50**(4): 101–5.

19 Sampson FC, Hayward A, Evans G, *et al.* Functional benefits and cost/benefit analysis of continuous intrathecal baclofen infusion for the management of severe spasticity. *J Neurosurg.* 2002; **96**(6): 1052–7.

20 Boviatsis EJ, Kouyialis AT, Korfias S, *et al.* Functional outcome of intrathecal baclofen administration for severe spasticity. *Clin Neurol Neurosurg.* 2005; **107**(4): 289–95.

21 Wade DT, Robson P, House H, *et al.* A preliminary controlled study to determine whether whole-plant cannabis extracts can improve intractable neurogenic symptoms. *Clin Rehabil.* 2003; **17**: 21–9.

22 Zajicek J, Fox P, Sanders H, *et al.* Cannabinoids for treatment of spasticity and other symptoms related to multiple sclerosis (CAMS study): multicentre randomised placebo-controlled trial. *Lancet.* 2003; **362**: 1517–26.

23 Smith PF. Cannabinoids in the treatment of pain and spasticity in multiple sclerosis. *Curr Opin Investig Drugs.* 2002; **3**(6): 859–64.

24 Pullman SC, Green P, Pahn S, *et al.* Approach to the treatment of limb disorders with botulinum toxin A: experience with 187 patients. *Arch Neurol.* 1996; **53**: 617–24.

25 Sheffield JK, Jankovic J. Botulinum toxin in the treatment of tremors, dystonias, sialorrhea and other symptoms associated with Parkinson's disease. *Expert Rev Neurother.* 2007; **7**(6): 637–47.

26 Brin MF, Lyons KE, Doucette J, *et al.* A randomised, double masked, controlled trial of botulinum toxin type A in essential hand tremor. *Neurol.* 2001; **56**: 1523–8.

27 Schneider SA, Edwards MJ, Cordivari C, *et al.* Botulinum toxin A may be efficacious as treatment for jaw tremor in Parkinson's disease. *Mov Disord.* 2006; **21**(10): 1722–4.

28 Limousin P, Memim B, Pollak B. Treatment of dystonia occurring in parkinsonism by botulinum toxin. *Eur Neurol.* 1997; **37**: 66–7.

29 Pacchetti C, Albani G, Martignoni E, *et al.* 'Off' painful dystonia in Parkinson's disease treated with botulinum toxin. *Mov Disord.* 1995; **10**(3): 333–6.

30 Costa J, Espirito-Santo C, Borges A, *et al.* Botulinum toxin type B for cervical dystonia. *Cochrane Database Syst Rev.* 2005; **1**: CD004315.

31 Costa J, Espirito-Santo C, Borges A, *et al.* Botulinum toxin type A for cervical dystonia. *Cochrane Database Syst Rev.* 2005; **1**: CD003633.

32 Costa J, Borges A, Espirito-Santo C. Botulinum toxin type A versus botulinum toxin type B for cervical dystonia. *Cochrane Database Syst Rev.* 2005; **1**: CD004314.

33 Bonelli RM, Wenning GK. Pharmacological management of Huntington's disease: an evidence-based review. *Curr Pharm Des.* 2006; **12**(21): 2701–20.

34 Adam OR, Jankovic J. Symptomatic treatment of Huntington disease. *Neurotherapeutics.* 2008; **5**(2): 181–97.

35 Huntington Study Group. Tetrabenazine as antichorea therapy in Huntington disease: a randomized controlled trial. *Neurol.* 2006; **66**: 366–72.

36 Bausewein C, Booth S, Gysels M, *et al.* Non-pharmacological interventions for breathlessness in advanced stages of malignant and non-malignant diseases. *Cochrane Database Syst Rev.* 2008; **2**: CD005623.

37 Jennings AL, Davies AN, Higgins JPT, *et al.* Opioids for the palliation of breathlessness in terminal illness. *Cochrane Database Syst Rev.* 2001; 4: CD002066.

38 Mitchell JD, Borasio GD. Amyotrophic lateral sclerosis. *Lancet.* 2007; **369**(9578): 2031–41.

39 Lyall RA, Moxham J, Leigh PN. Dyspnoea. In: Oliver D, Borasio GD, Walsh D, editors. *Palliative Care in Amyotrophic Lateral Sclerosis.* Oxford: Oxford University Press; 2000. pp. 43–56.

40 Chen R, Grand'Maison F, Strong MJ, *et al.* MND presenting as acute respiratory failure: a clinical and pathological study. *J Neurol Neurosurg Psychiatry.* 1996; **60**: 455–8.

41 Lyall RA, Donaldson N, Polkey MI, *et al.* Respiratory muscle strength and ventilatory failure in ALS. *Brain.* 2001; **124**: 2000–13.

42 Leigh PN, Abrahams S, Al-Chalabi A, *et al.* The management of motor neurone disease. *J Neurol Neurosurg Psychiatry.* 2003; **74**: 32–47.

43 Bourke SC, Tomlinson M, Williams TL, *et al.* Effects of non-invasive ventilation on survival and quality of life in patients with amyotrophic lateral sclerosis: a randomised controlled trial. *Lancet Neurol.* 2006; **5**: 140–7.

44 Bradley MD, Orrell RW, Clarke J, *et al.* Outcome of ventilatory support for acute respiratory failure in motor neurone disease. *J Neurol Neurosurg Psychiatry.* 2002; **72**: 752–6.

45 Hadjikoutis S, Eccles R, Wiles CM. Coughing and choking in motor neuron disease. *J Neurol Neurosurg Psychiatry.* 2000; **68**: 601–4.

46 Gdynia H-J, Kassubek J, Sperfeld A-D. Laryngospasm in neurological diseases. *Neurocrit Care.* 2006; **4**: 163–7.

47 Worwood A, Leigh PN. Indicators and prevalence of malnutrition in MND. *Eur Neurol.* 1998; **40**: 159–63.

48 Mazzini L, Corra T, Zaccala M, *et al.* Percutaneous endoscopic gastrostomy and enteral nutrition in amyotrophic lateral sclerosis. *J Neurol.* 1995; **242**: 695–8.

49 Bagheri H, Damase-Michel C, Lapeyre-Mestre M, *et al.* A study of salivary secretion in Parkinson's disease. *Clin Neuropharmacol.* 1999; **22**: 213–15.

50 Kalf JG, Smit AM, Bloem BR, *et al.* Impact of drooling in Parkinson's disease. *J Neurol.* 2007; **254**(9): 1227–32.

51 Marks L, Turner K, O'Sullivan J, *et al.* Drooling in Parkinson's disease: a novel speech and language therapy intervention. *Int J Lang Commun Disord.* 2001; **36**(Suppl.): S282–7.

52 Jongerius PH, van Teil P, van Limbeek J, *et al.* A systematic review for evidence of efficacy of anticholinergic drugs to treat drooling. *Arch Dis Child.* 2003; **88**(10): 911–14.

53 Lewis DW, Fontana C, Mehallick LK, *et al.* Transdermal scopolamine for reduction of drooling in developmentally delayed children. *Dev Med Child Neurol.* 1994; **36**: 484–6.

54 Brodtkorb E, Wyzocka-Bakowska MM, Lillevold PE, *et al.* Transdermal scopolamine in drooling. *J Ment Defic Res.* 1988; **32**(3): 233–7.

55 Al-Memar AY, Roy D, Powel A. Treatment with atropine sulphate 1% drops in the management of bulbar MND. *J Neurol Neurosurg Psychiatry.* 1998; **64**: 704.

56 Hyson HC, Johnson AM, Jog MS. Sublingual atropine for sialorrhea secondary to parkinsonism: a pilot study. *Mov Disord.* 2002; **17**(6): 1318–20.

57 Blasco PA, Stansbury JCK. Glycopyrrolate treatment of chronic drooling. *Arch Pediatr Adolesc Med.* 1996; **150**: 932–5.

58 Bachrach SJ, Walter RS, Trzeinski K. Use of glycopyrrolate and other cholinergic medications for sialorrhea in children with cerebral palsy. *Clin Pediatr.* 1998; **37**: 485–90.

59 Stern LM. Preliminary study of glycopyrrolate in the management of drooling. *J Paedriatr Child Health.* 1997; **33**: 52–4.

60 Mier RJ, Bachrach SJ, Lakin RC, *et al.* Treatment of sialorrhea with glycopyrrolate: a double-blind, dose-ranging study. *Arch Pediatr Adolesc Med.* 2000; **154**(12): 1214–18.

61 Strutt R, Fardell B, Chye R. Nebulized glycopyrrolate for drooling in a motor neuron patient. *J Pain Symptom Manage.* 2002; **23**(1): 2–3.

62 Camp-Bruno JA, Winsberg BG, Green-Parsons AR, *et al.* Efficacy of benztropine therapy for drooling. *Dev Med Child Neurol.* 1989; **31**(3): 309–19.

63 Reddihough D, Johnson H, Staples M, *et al.* Use of benzhexol hydrochloride to control drooling of children with cerebral palsy. *Dev Med Child Neurol.* 1990; **32**: 985–9.

64 Thomsen TR, Galpern WR, Asante A, *et al.* Ipratropium bromide spray as treatment for sialorrhea in Parkinson's disease. *Mov Disord.* 2007; **22**(15): 2268–73.

65 Newall AR, Orser R, Hunt M. The control of oral secretions in bulbar ALS/MND. *J Neurol Sci.* 1996; **139**(Suppl.): S43–4.

66 Dogu O, Apaydin D, Sevim S, *et al.* Ultrasound-guided versus 'blind' intraparotid injections of botulinum toxin-A for the treatment of sialorrhoea in patients with Parkinson's disease. *Clin Neurol Neurosurg.* 2004; **106**(2): 93–6.

67 Lagalla G, Millevolte M, Capecci M, *et al.* Botulinum toxin type A for drooling in Parkinson's disease: a double-blind, randomized, placebo-controlled study. *Mov Disord.* 2006; **21**(5): 704–7.

68 Lipp A, Trottenberg T, Schink T, *et al.* A randomized trial of botulinum toxin A for treatment of drooling. *Neurol.* 2003; **61**(9): 1279–81.

69 Mancini F, Zangaglia R, Cristina S, *et al.* Double-blind, placebo-controlled study to evaluate the efficacy and safety of botulinum toxin type A in the treatment of drooling in parkinsonism. *Mov Disord.* 2003; **18**(6): 685–8.

70 Ondo WG, Hunter C, Moore W. A double-blind placebo-controlled trial of botulinum toxin B for sialorrhea in Parkinson's disease. *Neurol.* 2004; **62**(1): 37–40.

71 Contarino MF, Pompili M, Tittoto P, *et al.* Botulinum B ultrasound guided injections for sialorrhea in amyotrophic lateral sclerosis and Parkinson's disease. *Parkinsonism Relat Disord.* 2007; **13**(5): 299–303.

72 Jongerius PH, Rotteveel JJ, van Limbeek J, *et al.* Botulinum toxin effect on salivary flow rate in children with cerebral palsy. *Neurol.* 2004; **63**(8): 1371–5.

73 Andersen PM, Gronberg H, Franzen L, *et al.* External radiation of the parotid glands significantly reduces drooling in patients with motor neurone disease and bulbar paresis. *J Neurol Sci.* 2001; **191**: 111–14.

74 Stalpers LJ, Moser EC. Results of radiotherapy for drooling in amyotrophic lateral sclerosis. *Neurol.* 2002; **58**: 1308.

75 Borg M, Hirst F. The role of radiation therapy in the management of sialorrhea. *Int J Radiat Oncol Biol Phys.* 1998; **41**: 1113–19.

76 Hockstein NG, Samadi DS, Gendron K, *et al*. Sialorrhea management challenge. *Am Fam Physician*. 2004; **69**(11): 2628–34.

77 Toepfer M, Folwaczny C, Klauser A, *et al*. Gastrointestinal dysfunction in amyotrophic lateral sclerosis. *Amyotroph Lateral Scler Other Motor Neuron Disord*. 1999; **1**(1): 15–19.

78 Kirkwood SC, Su JL, Conneally P, *et al*. Progression of symptoms in the early and middle stages of Huntington disease. *Arch Neurol*. 2001; **58**(2): 273–8.

79 Frontoni M, Giubilei F. Autonomic dysfunction in MS. *Int MSJ*. 1999; **6**(3): 79–87.

80 Fredrikson S. Nasal spray desmopressin treatment of bladder dysfunction in patients with multiple sclerosis. *Acta Neurol Scand*. 1996; **94**: 31–4.

81 Allain H, Schuck S, Mauduit N. Depression in Parkinson's disease. *BMJ*. 2000; **320**: 1287–8.

82 Kurt A, Nijboer F, Matuz T, *et al*. Depression and anxiety in individuals with amyotrophic lateral sclerosis: epidemiology and management. *CNS Drugs*. 2007; **21**(4): 279–91.

83 Sadovnick AD, Remick RA, Allen J, *et al*. Depression and multiple sclerosis. *Neurol*. 1996; **46**(3): 628–32.

84 National Institute for Health and Clinical Excellence. *Management of Multiple Sclerosis in Primary and Secondary Care: NICE guideline 8*. London: NICE; 2003. www.nice.org. uk/Guidance/CG8

85 Abrahams S, Goldstein LH, Al Chalabi A, *et al*. Relation between cognitive dysfunction and pseudobulbar palsy in amyotrophic lateral sclerosis. *J Neurol Neurosurg Psychiatry*. 1997; **62**: 464–72.

86 Figved N, Klevan G, Myhr KM, *et al*. Neuropsychiatric symptoms in patients with multiple sclerosis. *Acta Psychiatr Scand*. 2005; **112**(6): 463–8.

87 Feinstein A, Feinstein K, Gray T, *et al*. Prevalence and neurobehavioral correlates of pathological laughing and crying in multiple sclerosis. *Arch Neurol*. 1997; **54**(9): 1116–21.

88 Gallagher JP. Pathologic laughter and crying in amytrophic lateral sclerosis: a search for their origin. *Acta Neurol Scand*. 1989; **80**: 114–17.

89 Iannaccone S, Ferini-Strambi L. Pharmacologic treatment of emotional lability. *Clin Neuropharmacol*. 1996; **19**(6): 532–5.

90 Panitch HS, Thisted RA, Smith RA, *et al*. Randomized, controlled trial of dextromethorphan/quinidine for pseudobulbar affect in multiple sclerosis. *Ann Neurol*. 2006; **59**(5): 780–7.

91 Adler CH, Caviness JN, Hentz JG, *et al*. Randomized trial of modafinil for treating subjective daytime sleepiness in patients with Parkinson's disease. *Mov Disord*. 2003; **18**: 287–93.

92 Högl B, Saletu M, Brandauer E, *et al*. Modafinil for the treatment of daytime sleepiness in Parkinson's disease: a double-blind, randomized, crossover, placebo-controlled polygraphic trial. *Sleep*. 2002; **25**: 905–9.

93 Havlikova E, Rosenberger J, Nagyova I, *et al*. Clinical and psychosocial factors associated with fatigue in patients with Parkinson's disease. *Parkinsonism Relat Disord*. 2008; **14**(3): 187–92.

94 Rees PM, Fowler CJ, Maas CP. Sexual function in men and women with neurological disorders. *Lancet*. 2007; **369**(9560): 512–25.

95 Fowler CJ. The cause and management of bladder, sexual and bowel symptoms in multiple sclerosis. *Baillieres Clin Neurol.* 1997; **6**(3): 447–66.

96 Swinn L, Schrag A, Viswanathan R, *et al.* Sweating dysfunction in Parkinson's disease. *Mov Disord.* 2003; **18**(12): 1459–63.

97 Schestatsky P, Valls-Sole J, Ehlers JA, *et al.* Hyperhidrosis in Parkinson's disease. *Mov Disord.* 2006; **21**(10): 1744–8.

98 Santos-Bento M, de Carvalho M, Evangelista T, *et al.* Sympathetic sudomotor function and amyotrophic lateral sclerosis. *Amyotroph Lateral Scler Other Motor Neuron Disord.* 2001; **2**(2): 105–8.

99 Beck M, Giess R, Magnus T, *et al.* Progressive sudomotor dysfunction in amyotrophic lateral sclerosis. *J Neurosurg Psychiatry.* 2002; **73**(1): 68–70.

100 Wilson E, Elkan R, Seymour J, *et al.* A UK literature review of progressive long-term neurological conditions. *Br J Community Nurs.* 2008; **13**(5): 206, 208–12.

CHAPTER 5

Challenges to communication

Lorraine Dixon, Craig Maddock and Kim Wilcox

POLICY CONTEXT

Communication is a continual challenge in the care of patients with life limiting illness at the end of life. Recent political drives aim to improve communication within health and social care and help practitioners to establish what is meant by best practice. Specifically, there has been a move to address and improve quality of communication between health and social care professionals and with people with palliative and end of life care needs.[1] This has been a fundamental focus of the Department of Health's End of Life Care Strategy.[2] Effective communication is a core principle of the palliative care approach, with an emphasis on open and sensitive communication and extending this to patients, informal carers and professional colleagues.[3] The National Service Framework for Long-term (Neurological) Conditions is no exception in applying this principle, with recommendations throughout the document to communicate effectively.[4] It encourages a number of quick wins to improve care of the neurological patient, all based on the need for solid communication. For example:

➤ sharing examples of good practice
➤ improving lines of multi-agency communication
➤ involving users in communicating issues and initiating change
➤ recommending the appointment of practitioners with specialist skills and knowledge to communicate with patients, their families and professionals.

This is fundamentally changing a culture of practice, moving from a reliance on motivated individuals to drive the need for better communication towards encouraging organisational responsibility and accountability for improving communication. Organisational commitment is essential if individual examples of good practice are to be progressed and adapted as a common practice. There is evidence also that the context in which practitioners operate plays a significant role in the way they communicate: specifically the culture of the environment; the personalities involved; the religious beliefs of the practitioners; and their attitudes to death, rather than having specific education on communication.[5]

Maintaining effective communication is a constant challenge for all health and social care practitioners and organisations, irrespective of their role or practice setting. It is recognised that poor communication leads to a significant number of complaints each year. The Healthcare Commission's recent survey of complaints within the NHS highlighted poor communication as one of the contributory factors that significantly reduces the quality of care given at the end of life.[6] Poor communication rarely arises from intentional action by the practitioner to communicate badly; it is more likely to result from a medical model approach to communication which focuses on pathological disease and history taking at the expense of understanding the highly individual needs and perspectives of the patient.[7]

Professionals may avoid having difficult conversations for a number of different reasons.

➤ they are inhibited by their own agenda
➤ fear of blame
➤ lack of confidence in their own ability
➤ perceived lack of time
➤ poor organisational skill
➤ fear of getting a reaction that they lack confidence in dealing with
➤ recognising their own boundaries
➤ feeling they do not have the authority to respond.[8]

Patients report examples of good communication which stem from practitioners using an approach that has a holistic process, accurate content – one where perceptual skills of the practitioner are evident.[9] The evidence demonstrates the need for practitioners to develop their communication and interpersonal skills in order to facilitate the process of communication with the patient rather than engaging in blocking and distancing tactics that prevent effective dialogue.[10]

The Department of Health identified communication as a core skill for its workforce within the Knowledge and Skills Framework (KSF).[11] The KSF is essentially a development tool to enable staff within the NHS to progress through pay bands. It has however provided the workforce with explicit guidance as to what is expected within their role. The communication dimension applicable to all roles relates to effective communication in whatever form (e.g. verbal, non verbal and written) it takes place.[12] Four levels were identified.

1 Communicate with a limited range of people on day to day matters.
2 Communicate with a range of people on a range of matters.

3 Develop and maintain communication with people about difficult matters and/or in difficult situations.
4 Develop and maintain communication with people on complex matters, issues and ideas and/or in complex situations.

Each level provides key indicators and examples for practical applications . This provides the practitioner and employer with a baseline and standards which can be measured, thus enabling areas of poor practice to be identified and improved. It has the potential to provide clarity of expectation for patients and professionals. This chapter focuses on the evidence, skills and knowledge that are associated with Levels 3 and 4. It provides a synopsis of the recent policy developments which strive to improve communication. It is not an exhaustive or complete review of communication in this area of practice but it also aims to provide the individual with the opportunity to consider the evidence and reflect on their practice with respect to the following.

➤ Identifying best practice for communication with people with palliative and end of life care needs
➤ Outlining the challenges of applying best communication practice in the care of people affected by progressive long-term neurological conditions (PLTNCs)
➤ Looking at specific situations and providing guidance for best practice in relation to team working and coordination; disclosure of diagnosis; advance care planning; and assessment of capacity.

EVIDENCE BASE FOR BEST PRACTICE FOR COMMUNICATION

The importance of communication and counselling is referred to extensively within the literature and is regularly cited as something that requires improvement.[13] It features regularly in education programmes with taught coverage of practical descriptors to assist practitioners' skill and knowledge of communication. However, a systematic Cochrane Review of the literature surrounding communication in cancer care suggested that communication skills do not reliably improve with experience, despite considerable effort dedicated to courses improving communication skills for health professionals.[14] It recommended that evaluation of courses is vitally important to demonstrate evidence based teaching and practice, and to acquire a better understanding of what is needed to ensure a sustained improvement in communication.

The lack of conclusive evidence provides a significant challenge to employers with there being no consistent solution to ensure communication skills training programmes are effective and influence patients' outcomes. There is evidence that skills and knowledge may improve practice but no guarantee that it is sustained or that behaviours are altered and improved.[15] Current programmes rely on the individual practitioner to be sufficiently self aware to take time to develop their knowledge and skills. The communication skills training programmes currently in existence are primarily focused around promoting self awareness in practitioners; exploration of communication behaviours (e.g. verbal, non verbal and paralinguistic with respect to the positive and negative impact on patient interaction); and learning through techniques (e.g. role play where there is the opportunity to simulate and practice communication skills).[16] None of the existing programmes are specific to the issues of dealing with PLTNCs.

As palliative care has developed as a specialty it has sought to support patients and their families with complex and challenging decisions, using explicit techniques for handling difficult conversations and removing professional fear of challenging communication. Regardless of the approach to decision making, the success of the approach is dependent on the effectiveness of the communication activities. Box 5.1 is adapted from work undertaken with people with intellectual disabilities and captures the communication skills, aptitude and knowledge that practitioners should have to be able to communicate effectively.[17]

BOX 5.1 Effective practitioner communication

Practitioners should be able to:
- provide care that is accessible to people with communication difficulties;
- be aware of potential communication difficulties and the skills required to minimise such barriers to effective reciprocal communication;
- be aware of the range of assessment tools available to measure the distress, that have a particular emphasis on limited verbal or cognitive abilities;
- conduct appropriate holistic palliative care assessments of the patients and their families in relation to their physical, psychological, social, spiritual and informational needs;
- recognise and understand when and how to seek advice or refer to a specialist palliative care service and other agencies;
- work in collaboration with the specialist palliative care service and others to meet the needs of the patient with a life limiting illness;
- recognise their own skill deficit and make appropriate referrals.

Communication becomes complex for a number of different reasons.
➤ lack of time
➤ lack of knowledge or skills of the practitioner concerned
➤ patient need and point in disease trajectory
➤ environment
➤ misunderstanding and differing perception.

This is by no means an exhaustive list but it illustrates the challenges for practitioners in managing often multiple and constantly changing variables.

CHALLENGES OF APPLYING BEST PRACTICE IN THE CARE OF PLTNCs

Care of patients affected by PLTNCs provides a unique set of challenges for health and social care professionals and carers at the end of life. This often presents a complex set of needs, with multiple agencies involved, all aiming to manage the needs through integrated packages of health and social care. Effective professional communication is essential to facilitate coordination and execution of care in response to patient need. Patients with acquired neurological conditions develop their verbal communication and literacy capabilities as typical speakers and writers, but then gradually or suddenly lose some or all of their ability due to their neurological condition.[18] Support for the individual, their family and carers to manage the adjustment and impact on daily living may require creative and thorough care planning. Recognition of the potential physical reasons why communication can be impaired for services users with progressive long-term conditions is important.[19] The following are brief descriptors of the key physical factors that arise from some neurological conditions.

Cognitive impairment. The potential changes in cognition due to neurological conditions include slower processing, reduced short-term memory, mental capacity and difficulty in maintaining the topic or any length of conversation.[20]

Lip function. Muscles in the lips and cheeks can be affected by diseases such as motor neurone disease or cerebral vascular accident. Changes in the muscles can make it difficult for the patient to produce the right shape with their mouth. A small change in shape can result in the pronunciation of the word being incorrect and difficult for the listener to distinguish.

Soft palate and pharyngeal function. As with the lips, the soft palate and pharynx have a role in influencing the sound produced. Where function of the area is compromised the change in sounds may result in sounds becoming unintelligible. The sounds may become laboured and blurred.

Tongue function. Impaired tongue function is of particular significance for patients with amyotrophic lateral sclerosis, with a reduction of the sounds produced and, as the disease progresses, speech becomes slurred and incomprehensible.

Laryngeal function. The larynx and vocal cords provide the capacity to speak. Weakness in the vocal cords is a common problem which can inhibit communication. Changes in the lower and upper motor neurone function can influence the movement of the vocal cords, resulting in change of pitch, tone and projection of voice.

Respiratory function. A compromised respiratory system can affect an individual's ability to communicate. To speak, a certain amount of lung capacity is required. Changes in respiratory function can influence speech by altering tone, rhythm, intonation and volume. Where respiratory function is compromised due to infection this can affect the ability to communicate. Weakness or injury in the spinal cord resulting in upper or lower motor neurone loss may affect the strength of respirations making it difficult for patients to raise sufficient volume in their voice to be heard, or to speak more than a few words with each breath.[21]

Body posture. The posture of the body can also affect the patient's ability to communicate. They may be physically unable to project their voice due to poor posture or get tired maintaining a posture that enables them to communicate easily. Posture may exacerbate the physical problems mentioned above.

Fatigue. Fatigue can be a related symptom of progressive neurological conditions. Coping with associated symptoms like dysphasia can exhaust the patient, leaving them with little energy to engage in communication.

Pathological laughing and crying. Physical damage or disease in some neurological conditions can alter neurological function and cause uncontrollable laughing or crying, both of which can inhibit effective communication.

Any of the above can influence the patient's ability to communicate effectively, to convey their needs, to socialise and to remain independent.

GUIDANCE FOR BEST PRACTICE

The principles of good communication are common across all situations. They are dependent on the patient being able to hear, see and speak. Each PLTNC may vary in how it affects these systems, discussed earlier in the chapter. It should not be assumed that all patients with a PLTNC will be able to communicate in the same way; this makes it necessary to utilise an individualistic and creative approach to communication. There are key principles to guiding communication at the end of life:[22]

➤ be honest and truthful
➤ ask about patient values and goals
➤ help explore options within the context of their values and goals
➤ encourage questions
➤ ask yourself, 'What would I do if this were my family member?'
➤ take time to listen
➤ don't avoid difficult conversations, but ask for assistance if it is beyond your confidence and ability
➤ be prepared before starting the conversation.

TEAM WORKING AND COORDINATION

Patients come into contact with a vast number of practitioners in their disease trajectory. The complexities of PLTNCs require effective and coordinated professional communication. Use of a key worker who has a rapport with the patient can help to minimise unnecessary repetition, aid communication and avoid embarrassing misunderstanding. Establishing a common set of documentation for professionals and carers to record communication can help conversations to move on, rather than cover the same ground. The literature suggests that teams require self analysis, empathy and flexibility to collaborate effectively,[23] which demands clear direction and a supportive and safe environment to raise and debate concerns.[24] Where communication is particularly challenging, the involvement of an expert practitioner familiar with the set of problems inhibiting the communication can be helpful. Early referral to speech and language therapists (SALTs) is important in the early stages of some long-term neurological conditions, to offer advice and establish strategies to cope with and manage the communication difficulties before speech becomes an obvious problem. Through the discussions to establish strategies there is also opportunity to discuss how things may change in the future and therefore prepare in advance for deterioration of the physical or mental ability to communicate.

DISCLOSURE OF DIAGNOSIS

Studies surrounding the disclosure of diagnosis to cancer patients reveal that nurses were opposed to withholding diagnosis at the wish of relatives, and that they found deception was difficult to maintain and produced distressing consequences for patients and their families.[25] Fear of talking about death and the perceived impact on the patient were usually the motivations for relatives wishing to protect their loved ones.[26] Historically, there has been an acceptance of this paternalistic approach which has been challenged as healthcare practice has become increasingly more aware of the complexity of ethical decision making. There are some principles that should be applied to disclosure of diagnosis or prognosis:
➤ approach disclosure in a sensitive and positive manner
➤ provide timely and appropriate support for the individual
➤ early sharing of information
➤ collaboration of professionals and carers in supporting the
  patient.[27]

ADVANCE CARE PLANNING

Advance care planning is an important part of preventative healthcare,[28] which requires a sensitive and considered approach, such as the 4 Step Advance Care

Planning Process[29] (*see* Box 5.2). This is not without challenge, as highlighted by the Reality Check: 10 Barriers to Advance Care Planning (*see* Box 5.2).

BOX 5.2 4 Step Advance Care Planning Process and Reality Check

4 Step Advance Care Planning Process	**Reality Check: 10 Barriers to Advance Care Planning**
1 Presenting the topic	1 Patient and provider reluctance
2 Facilitating discussion	2 Time constraints
3 Completing and documenting the advance directive	3 Assumptions
	4 Denial and procrastination
4 Reviewing and updating documents	5 Unrealistic expectations
	6 Delaying until a crisis
	7 Discomfort with palliative care planning
	8 Lack of documentation
	9 Cultural and health system barriers
	10 Patient readiness

Planning care where the patient has impaired verbal communication can be challenging. There are a number of tools available to assist with assessment, e.g. the disability distress tool,[30] which can help in approaching the assessment in a systematic and detailed manner. Tools should however be used with caution and constantly reviewed as to their appropriateness and reliability for the purpose that that are being used for.

ASSESSMENT OF CAPACITY

The UK Mental Capacity Act (MCA) aimed to improve the quality and experience of care for patients whose capacity to make decisions for themselves and about their own care is impaired in some way.[31] It is particularly pertinent where the patient has not had the opportunity to go through the advance care planning process to make decisions in advance of their mental capacity being compromised by their PLTNC. Where mental capacity is variable the supportive role of the practitioner in working to optimise the effectiveness of the communication for patients is essential to facilitate effective decision making. This may involve:

➤ scheduling the communication after a period of rest or at the particular time of day when the patient is most able to manage communication

➤ creating protected time within the day to enable the communication to progress at a speed acceptable to the patient

➤ ensuring the communication is carried out in a suitable environment free from distraction
➤ utilising strategies to facilitate communication and aid decision making that are tailored to the individual's need.

The MCA suggests that a patient does not have the mental capacity to make the decision if he/she is unable to:
a. understand the information relevant to the decision
b. retain the information
c. use or weigh that information as part of the process of making the decision; or
d. communicate his decision (whether by talking, using sign language or any other means).[34]

The practitioner under these circumstances must make the judgement call as to whether or not the patient is to be regarded as unable to understand the information relevant to a decision or if he is able to understand an explanation of it given to him in a way that is appropriate to his circumstances (using simple language, visual aids or any other means). Where the patient is able to retain the information relevant to a decision for a short period only it does not prevent him from being regarded as able to make the decision.[34] The practitioner must attempt to convey the information relevant to a decision, inclusive of information regarding the reasonably foreseeable consequences of deciding one way or another, or failing to make the decision.[34] Where possible, families and carers should be engaged in the process.

In a joint statement by the Commission for Social Care Inspection, Healthcare Commission, and Mental Health Act Commission, it is made clear that organisations have a responsibility and are accountable for ensuring that practitioners working within health and social care have the necessary skills and knowledge to support decision making where mental capacity is compromised for an individual.[35] Systems of clinical governance should be in place to ensure mental capacity is appropriately considered in the provision of care. This may require the use of a tool to assess and monitor mental capacity in order to ensure a consistent approach is utilised in the application of the MCA.

The MCA has had profound implications for end of life decision making.[32] Where a patient is felt not to have the mental capacity to make a decision, someone else must make the decision on their behalf but in the patient's best interest.[33] 'Best interest' is when we make a decision for someone else and the practitioner or care team must ensure that the decision made is the best decision based on what is known about the patient and their unique circumstances. Where a 'best interest' decision is required a logical process should be followed.

1 Identification of who should be involved in the decision making process and identify a decision maker to lead the process.
2 Clear identification of the proposal and other treatment options.
3 Consideration of issues in preparation for discussion.
4 Meeting key stakeholders to discuss the proposal.[34]
5 Clear recording and documentation of decision made.

CASE EXAMPLE 5.1 Rachel

Rachel was a 61 year old woman diagnosed with multiple sclerosis 15 years earlier. She lived with her husband and son in a bungalow. She had been very active and enthusiastic about life. As her condition deteriorated she began to lose interest in the activities of daily living and became obsessive about her symptoms. She developed a fear of being alone which was exacerbated by her lifelong fear of the dark. She had heightened anxiety and sought constant reassurance and attention. When she was awake her attention seeking behaviour increased considerably. She ate little; her fluid input/output also diminished. Rachel's care had substantially increased and her demands on her husband became a prime consideration. The community team were finding her difficult to manage in the time they had within their caseload.

To facilitate broader communication a case conference was arranged including all of the practitioners involved in Rachel's care. This consisted of Rachel and her husband, her GP and district nurse, consultant psychiatrist and clinical psychologist, MS nurse consultant, a hospice support worker and an occupational therapist. Throughout the whole process leading up to and including the case conference Rachel had been fully involved in the choices and consented to the process taking place. The team also felt that although Rachel's husband had enduring power of attorney and despite Rachel's psychiatric history she had capacity to be involved in decisions regarding her future care.

The case conference enabled discussion about Rachel's future care and support for her husband. The psychiatrist and psychologist were able to help her identify strategies that had helped her to cope in the past and to share these with the community team and the day hospice. This enabled reinforcement of strategies following the case conference. Rachel was able to recognise through the discussion that her attention seeking behaviour was because she was frightened about the future. The openness of the discussion enabled Rachel to verbalise how she would like to be cared for in the future and to actively draw up an action plan with the practitioners that she felt happy with. Respite care via her weekly visit to the day hospice was continued and continuing healthcare funding was accessed to provide further care at home.

Case Example 5.1 highlights the importance of respecting the individual's mental capacity to be in control of their decision making. It also highlights the importance of team collaboration to pool resources in organising support. The opportunity for Rachel to communicate about her fears and anxieties was essential and helped in shaping the ongoing psychological support that she required.

CASE EXAMPLE 5.2 Jane

Jane was admitted to the hospice with cerebral metastases which had not responded to chemotherapy and exacerbated unpleasant neurological symptoms. She was only able to hear loud voices in one ear. She was also blind. Her mobility had gradually deteriorated over the previous few weeks; from being able to mobilise with assistance, to being bed bound. Initially upon admission she could move her arms, hands, head and shoulders, and she could make herself understood. She was desperate to return home but her husband and eldest daughter, who had been caring for her at home, were exhausted and feeling unable to cope. They had no special equipment and had not considered the option of an outside carer being employed to help them. As Jane's mobility worsened following the chemotherapy, the husband contacted the out of hours GP, who re-admitted Jane to the local acute hospital where she was assessed and transferred to the hospice for end of life care.

When Jane arrived, it was clear to everyone involved with her care that she was in charge. Her wish was to get home as quickly as possible. She accepted her prognosis was not good but was keen to look at any option which might improve her symptoms or extend her life. On the day of admission we began to plan for her discharge, as we knew that our window of opportunity was dependent upon Jane being well enough to make an ambulance journey home and her symptoms being sufficiently under control to be able to be managed at home.

Assessments of Jane had taken place prior to the weekly multidisciplinary team meeting (MDT). Present in the meeting were the medical staff, social worker, nurses, occupational therapist and physiotherapist. Reports from her husband, daughter, district nurse, and GP were also presented. Within the meeting the issues that might create a barrier to Jane's discharge home were discussed and a consensus reached. Potential solutions to overcome the problems were identified. The social worker took the lead coordinating the planning to get Jane home, as she had built a good rapport with Jane and her family. She also knew the community team supporting Jane well.

Following the MDT the social worker met with Jane, her family and the district nurse to present the potential package of support. The meeting took place at Jane's bedside. All those attending made a conscious effort to speak clearly, and sit on the side where she had better hearing.

- Information was shared to outline the support that could be offered and talk through the potential problems that might occur. Open discussion was had regarding the support for Jane, her husband and her daughter.
- The agreed plan of care was summarised and documented, with a copy of the plan given to Jane, her husband, the district nurse and a copy kept as a record in her notes.
- A plan regarding who would contact the services and personnel who would be supporting Jane's discharge.

By the following morning the whole team and Jane's family had the care package in place, and an ambulance booked for Jane's discharge home that evening. Jane's wish to die at home was about to be achieved. However, over the next 6 hours Jane became anxious about the discharge as she became uncomfortable with the reality of her desire to die at home. Following an intense period with Jane and her husband she finally made the decision to stay in the hospice. She expressed that it had been important for her to know it was possible to go home and that the support could be in place. All parties involved were satisfied that we had made every effort to support Jane's wishes and preferred place of care. Nobody felt disappointed or that their time had been wasted.

Case Example 5.2 also highlights the importance of team collaboration and the need to be flexible in supporting the patient's wishes, despite the considerable effort required to mobilise care to support her at home. The case illustrates that it is possible to organise care at home in a relatively short period of time. A significant learning point for the care team was that a patient's preferred place of care can change dependent on the situation at the time. For Jane the reality of facing a death at home became too much. Without effective communication her change in wishes may not have been realised in time.

CHALLENGES FOR THE FUTURE

Supporting someone during the last stages of their life is always difficult,[35] regardless of whether the communication is straightforward or has added complexity due to the physical challenges that a PLTNC can bring. Practitioners have an important role to play in the assessment of the individualised needs of the patient.[36] The important consideration is 'not what is said but what is understood'[37] as this will have a lasting impression on the patient and their families. The challenge for the future is to rise to the challenge of the recent political drives aiming to improve and sustain effective communication within health and social care, to help practitioners to establish what is meant by best practice, and ultimately to improve the delivery of care for patients and their families.

REFERENCES

1 Darzi A. *High Quality Care for All: NHS Next Stage Review final report.* London: TSO; 2008.

2 Department of Health. *End of Life Care Strategy: promoting high quality care for all adults at the end of life.* London: COI; 2008.

3 Wilkinson S, Mula C. Communication in care of the dying. In: Ellershaw J, Wilkinson S, editors. *Care of the Dying: a pathway to excellence.* Oxford: Oxford University Press; 2003. pp. 74–5.

4 Department of Health. *National Service Framework for Long-term (Neurological) Conditions.* London: COI; 2005.

5 Dunne K. Effective communication. *Nurs Stand.* 2005; **20**(13): 57–64.

6 Fellowes D, Wilkinson S, Moore P. Communications skills training for health care professionals working with cancer patients, their families and/or carers. *Cochrane Database Syst Rev.* 2004; 2: CD003751.

7 Jarrett N, Maslin-Prothero S. Communication, the patient and the palliative care team. In: Payne S, Seymour J, Ingleton C, editors. *Palliative Nursing: principles and evidence for practice.* Oxford: Oxford University Press; 2004. pp. 90–107.

8 Wilkinson S, op. cit.

9 Wilkinson S. Factors which influence how nurses communicate with cancer patients. *J Adv Nurs.* 1991; **16**: 677–88.

10 Ibid.

11 NHS Executive. *A Policy Framework for Commissioning Cancer Services: palliative care services.* EL (96)85. London: NHSE; 1996.

12 Ibid.

13 Ashurst A. Palliative care: effective communication. *Nursing & Residential Care.* 2007; **9**(2): 66–8.

14 Fellowes D, *et al.*, op. cit.

15 Ibid.

16 Silverman J, Kurtz S, Draper J. *Skills for Communicating with Patients.* 2nd ed. Oxford: Radcliffe Publishing; 2005.

17 Gauthier DM. Challenges and opportunities: communication near the end of life. *Medsurg Nurs.* 2008; **17**(5): 291–6.

18 Beukelmann DR, Fager S, Ball L, *et al.* AAC for adults with acquired neurological conditions: a review. *Augment Altern Commun.* 2007; **23**(3): 230–42.

19 Scott A, Foulsum M. Speech and language therapy. In: Oliver D, Borasio GD, Walsh D. *Palliative Care in Amyotrophic Lateral Sclerosis.* Oxford: Oxford University Press; 2000. pp. 117–32.

20 Guyon A. Assessments: speech and language therapy. *Nursing & Residential Care.* 2007; **9**(10): 486–9.

21 Murphy J. 'I prefer contact this close': perceptions of AAC by people with motor neurone disease and their communication partners. *AAC.* 2004; **20**(4): 259–71.

22 Maxfield CL, Pohl JM, Colling K. Advance directives: a guide for patient discussions. *Nurse Pract.* 2003; **28**(5): 38–47.

23 Dawson S. Interprofessional working: communication, collaboration . . . perspiration! *Int J Palliat Nurs.* 2007; **13**(10): 502–5.

24 Ibid.

25 Kendall S. Being asked not to tell: nurses' experiences of caring for cancer patients not told their diagnosis. *J Clin Nurs.* 2006. **15**: 1149–57.

26 Duffin C. Let's talk about death. *Nurs Older People.* 2008; **20**(6): 6–7.

27 Monaghan C, Begley A. Dementia and disclosure: a dilemma in practice. *J Clin Nurs.* 2004; **13**(3a): 22–9.

28 Maxfield CL, *et al.*, op. cit.

29 Foster J, Turner M. Implications of the Mental Capacity Act 2005 on advanced care planning at the end of life. *Nurs Stand.* 2007; **22**(2): 35–9.

30 Ibid.

31 Ashurst A. Palliative care: effective communication. *Nursing & Residential Care.* 2007; **9**(2): 66–8.

32 Ibid.

33 Cooley C. Communication is the key to care. *Int J Palliat Nurs.* 2006; **12**(10): 479–84.

34 Office of Public Sector Information. *Mental Capacity Act 2005.* Available at: www. opsi.gov.uk/ACTS/acts2005/ukpga_20050009_en_2 (accessed 16 February 2009).

35 Mental Capacity Act: Joint Statement by the Commission for Social Care Inspection, Healthcare Commission, Mental Health Act Commission. 2008. Available at: www. carestandards.org.uk/docs/20080116%20Joint%20CSCI%20HC%20MHAC%20 %20Statement%20on%20MCA%20007-081.doc (accessed 16 February 2009).

CHAPTER 6

Patients and families

Eleanor Wilson

INTRODUCTION

The aim of this chapter is to give an insight into the experiences of people (both patients and family caregivers) living with a progressive long-term neurological condition (PLTNC), particularly in relation to service access and delivery, and those factors that promote or constrain their quality of life. There is currently limited research and published discussion focusing on the personal experiences of those affected by a PLTNC. Hence a case study from the author's doctoral research which explores the care needs of people affected by Huntington's disease (HD) is used to illustrate some of the issues raised (pseudonyms are used throughout in order to maintain anonymity).

CONTEXT OF CARE

In the UK, the majority of care for people living with PLTNCs is community based, usually delivered in a person's home. This reflects, on the one hand, a policy emphasis on the promotion of community based care[1,2] and, on the other, the scarce availability of inpatient or long-term care sites with the expertise needed to provide care for people with the complex physical and mental impairments associated with PLTNCs. The published literature relating to general issues in community based service provision tends to make particular reference to the needs of people with Parkinson's disease (PD) and multiple sclerosis (MS). Discussions which relate specifically to palliative and end of life care service provision are found in the field of motor neurone disease (MND) care, with the majority of UK publications emerging from two leading hospices which have a special interest in MND: St Christopher's, London[3,4] and Wisdom Hospice, Kent,[5-7] often in collaboration with the MND Association.[8,9]

Wilson, *et al.* provide a review of the UK literature on community care service provision,[10] highlighting the key challenges of uneven coverage and lack of flexibility. The review shows that, in line with current policy trends, multidisciplinary care delivery is considered essential,[1] with communication and coordination of multidisciplinary teams regarded as complex yet vital for timely, flexible and appropriate care to be delivered to those in need. A key theme relates to the invaluable contribution to a person's palliative and end of life care of each multidisciplinary team member, many of whom will have been involved in care delivery for a considerable time and who are thus in a position to guide and support the delivery of such care.[11] The review identifies both the high value that patients and carers place on the role of 'key workers' as coordinators of care and information across the disease trajectory and the importance of maximising a person's potential for self managed care where this is possible.[12] Further, an emphasis is placed on the need for professional care staff to work in partnership with family caregivers who in many cases will have developed significant expertise in providing care and support to their family member. For example, Lees, *et al.* argue, in their examination of palliative care delivery in PD, that family carers who endure significant impact on their own lives must be considered not only as a source of support, guidance and advice but as a key part of the wider multidisciplinary team.[11]

LIVING WITH A PLTNC

As illustrated in other chapters, people with PLTNCs live with and manage a wide range of complex physical and psychiatric symptoms throughout the course of their illness. They will experience continuous losses over time and become increasingly dependent on other people for physical care. For example, in an interview based study exploring the experiences of people severely affected by MS, Edmonds, *et al.*[13] identify three key areas of loss: a person's physical abilities, their independence and relationships. Each of these elements is intrinsically linked and has influences which extend into the family and wider social network surrounding the person with the neurological condition.

With neurological disease progression, increasing cognitive impairment means that a person may lose the ability to instigate or maintain tasks, have reduced short-term memory, or become easily agitated.[14] Physical deficits such as inability to control movements, limb weakness, and impaired speech and swallowing all add to a continuum of losses over time.[13,15,16] These cumulate into a loss of independence, thus changing relationships with spouses, children, other family and friends.[17,18] The husband or wife becomes a 'carer', children begin to look after a parent and friends are needed to help with chores and provide emotional support.

IMPACT ON FAMILY

There is now an increasing body of research accessing the experience of living with and caring for someone with a PLTNC. Family carers have a fundamental and essential role in providing daily long-term care, the importance of which has tended to be under recognised, as Carter, *et al.*[19] acknowledge in their study of spousal carers living with a person who has PD:

> Families are the most valuable and also the most vulnerable resource we have . . .. With the diagnosis . . . comes the role of family caregiving. The work of caregiving is demanding and ever-changing, increasing as the disease progresses and disability becomes more pronounced.[19]

Family carers daily undertake both physical and emotional labour[20] as they manage not only the 24 hour care of another adult but also run a household, pay the bills, look after the children.[21] They may be facing the challenge of holding down a job while making difficult decisions about the care management and coordination which disrupt their working lives.[22] Moreover, they have to live with the emotional challenges which the caring role poses, sometimes while watching the person for whom they care change dramatically over time.[17] Family carers are not always able to live their own lives as they might otherwise wish: careers, social activities and hobbies are often curtailed or lost completely.[22]

With disease progression, relationships with the person with the PLTNC may shift to one based around the provision of nursing care and attention to bodily needs.[20] Twigg and Atkin[23] identify four main categories for the nature of physical care: personal care; the management of incontinence; medical and nursing care; and household tasks. Box 6.1 provides an overview of their book, *Carers Perceived*.

BOX 6.1 Overview of *Carers Perceived* by Twigg and Atkin[23]

> The authors describe how the intimate nature of personal care can be problematic:
>
>> Personal care involves touching, nakedness and contact with excreta . . . The meaning of personal care is mediated by relationship and gender. Different relationships imply different expectations, and what is acceptable for a parent to do for a child – even an adult child – may not be so in reverse. Breaching these boundaries may cause embarrassment and require special techniques of social distancing (p. 32).
>
> Twigg and Atkin identify that managing incontinence is one of the most stressful aspects of caring, for both the person cared for and the carer. Tasks can include managing colostomy bags, incontinence pads, catheters, accidents and additional laundry. Away from the home this can be particularly difficult. Nursing tasks

overlap with personal care but often extend into undertaking tasks that would be done by a trained nurse such as changing dressings, injections and supervising medication. Being comfortable with undertaking these types of tasks varies with different carers. Household tasks can also be problematic for carers who themselves are elderly or not in good health. Male carers are more likely to accept help with personal and nursing aspects of care, whereas women often struggle with the more traditionally male tasks.

In the case of HD, caregivers often have to deal with, and sensitively negotiate the avoidance of, aggressive and sometimes physically violent behaviours.[21,24,25] Where this no longer becomes possible to manage in the family home, long-term care is necessitated, particularly if children are involved and the home environment is no longer safe for them because of the person with HD. Tyler, *et al.*[21] report that violence is often a source of marriage breakdown in couples where one partner is affected by HD. More generally, across the diseases, deterioration of memory loss, understanding and ability to communicate are common, meaning that it is not just the person diagnosed with a PLTNC who experiences continuous loss, but also those close to them.

In a small qualitative study to explore and describe the experiences of family members of people with Huntington's disease, Semple[26] identified the main source of frustration for carers of people with HD to be directly related to a lack of community and family support. Carers perceived that they were given little choice in taking on the care giving role and yet they provided the majority of care to the person with HD. This gave rise to reports among family caregivers of feeling lonely, anxious, depressed and mistrusting professionals.

The strain associated with family care giving can result in crisis situations when the caregiver can no longer physically and emotionally manage the role.[21] In some instances the carer's own health is compromised:[22] for example, family caregivers of people with MND[27] have reported sleep deprivation as a common cause of continuous stress. Caring can also be potentially physically harmful, yet while professionals have training, equipment and health and safety recommendations to protect and guide them to carry out this work safely and effectively, in the domestic home the majority of carers have no such safeguards. Back pain, exhaustion and sleep deprivation[27] are all commonly reported. Older carers in particular may often find that their own health problems are exacerbated.

The positive effects of care giving are rarely reported, although Aubeeluck's work with the carers of people with HD has identified some elements of care that family caregivers considered to be positive, such as support from friends and relatives, the kindness of strangers, enjoying the small pleasures in life, spending time together.[28] Work by Nolan has also identified positive aspects to care giving and Box 6.2 provides an overview of Nolan's research.

BOX 6.2 Overview of 'Positive aspects of caring' by Nolan[29]

Nolan's work aims to highlight the range of satisfactions and rewards that carers may experience. He dispels the preconception that caring relationships are rarely reciprocal and that it is always necessary to focus on the relief of 'burden' by applying a therapeutic model delivered by professional 'experts'. Nolan argues that reciprocity is the basis of the satisfactions that can be derived from the caring role and shows that carers who identify positive aspects of caring, through focusing on reciprocal aspects of their experience, have higher levels of well-being and morale.

SERVICE INTERACTION

There is a body of research focusing on the views and opinions of health and social care professionals about service delivery to those affected by PLTNCs. While professional accounts of care can only provide indirect insight into the patient/carer experience, they do provide important information about care provision and highlight elements of best practice. Meeting the needs of those with PLTNCs can be challenging for health and social care professionals. The rarity of the diseases means that most GPs and district nurses, who will be called upon to deliver the majority of professional care, are likely to have little or no knowledge and experience of the conditions.

Among people with HD[30] and MND,[27] survey based research in Scotland highlights that appropriate and timely services are vital in sustaining care at home for a long as possible. The provision of respite care, financial aid, equipment and general advice are considered essential by both family carers and affected individuals in order to avoid crisis.[30] Among people with HD,[30] the urgent need to proactively plan service provision, involving where appropriate voluntary sector providers, is emphasised, since this is seen to help maintain independence, manage symptoms, reduce carer burden, and thus in the long-term present the most cost effective service delivery model.

Published research draws attention to the failure of traditional models of service provision to include patients and carers in decisions concerning their own care package. The importance of client centeredness is highlighted, through tailoring services individually in the light of clients' expressed wishes and needs, and ensuring flexibility in the light of changing needs.[31-6] Examples of innovative practice include services where patients can self refer.[32,37,38] In one study examining the self referral from the perspective of a community MS team,[37] patients were reported to be viewed as equal members of the multidisciplinary team, with a blurring of the boundaries between professional and user roles. In a study of a relapse service for people with MS,[38] it is reported that staff have developed education techniques to ensure that patients are able to self refer in an appropriate and timely manner. In a study of people's experiences of living with MND, Hughes, et al.[35] draw attention to the fact that a lack of patient and carer involvement results in a lost opportunity for professional education. They found that professionals involved in the care of people with MND often have little contact with, and little opportunity to learn from, their clients, and advocate the development of working groups of users and professionals to foster greater exchange of knowledge between the two groups.

In some cases, service delivery can be based on a model which extends beyond patient involvement or partnership in their care to self management by patients of their own care. This approach is exemplified by Lloyd's[39] report of patients with PD taking on the role of 'care managers', supported by professional knowledge, expertise and resources in order to manage their own situations. On the basis of her study of community care provision for people with PD, Lloyd[39] concludes that if service providers cease to treat care management solely as a professional activity and, instead, take seriously the patient as an untapped resource for managing their own situation, more effective accessing and targeting of services would ensue. Lloyd acknowledges that the most vulnerable may be unable to manage their own situation in this way, but argues that helping the majority of people to self manage would assist the early identification of the most vulnerable, and improve the targeting of those in need of intensive support.

In a study of professionally guided self care for people with MS, incorporating tailored discussions about self care using a self care booklet, O'Hara, et al.[31] also draw on the notion of 'self-management of care', arguing that this can enable patients to work effectively with professional staff and thus enable appropriate use of scarce resources such as community physiotherapy time.

EXPLORING THE CARE NEEDS OF THOSE AFFECTED BY HD: AN EXAMPLE OF ONGOING RESEARCH

Research exploring the care needs of those affected by HD is being undertaken as a doctoral study by the author at the University of Nottingham: the aim and objectives of the project are in Box 6.3. The project involves people affected by HD across three localities where the provision of care differs.

1   A multidisciplinary community team led by a HD specialist nurse, including a consultant, dietician and speech and language therapist.
2   A consultant clinic service with input from a Regional Care Advisor (RCA) from the Huntington's Disease Association (HDA).
3   A residential long-term nurse led specialist care centre.

BOX 6.3 An example of ongoing research on the care needs of those with HD

Aim

- To explore the care needs of those affected by HD.

Objectives

- To identify the supportive care needs of those diagnosed with HD.
- To identify the needs of informal carers/relatives caring for a person with HD.
- To gain an understanding of the issues encountered by health and social care professionals in delivering care to people with HD.
- To identify differences in the issues for care provision for those living in the family home and those in residential settings.

The study employs a collective case study approach with the person diagnosed with HD as the central component. Each case also incorporates a key family member and healthcare professional as identified by the person with HD. Staff at each location identify people who it may be possible to invite to take part in the study: a fundamental requirement is that they are able to understand the research and have a level of speech which would allow an interview to take place. The ongoing participation of each person with HD is assessed with regard to any changes in their capacity to consent during the research process and in cooperation with the person's family members and healthcare professionals. Interviews and observation methods are being used as data collection methods over a period of up to three years (between 2007–10).

CASE EXAMPLE 6.1 Sarah and Max

Sarah is 60 years old and is married to Max. Sarah and Max have two adult sons, both of whom are married; each with one young child of their own. Sarah was diagnosed with HD in 2001. In retrospect, Max reports his concerns that there had been something wrong for many years:

> *Max:* Well, she had, I mean I can go back to about 1970 . . . about 72/73. When you think about it now, it explains a lot.

There was no known history of HD in Sarah's family and everyone was shocked by her diagnosis. At the time the case study interviews were conducted, Sarah and Max's sons said that they did not wish to be tested for the presence of the mutated gene:

Max: No, no there was nothing in the family, nobody knew anything about it.

Sarah: It's to do with genes.

Max: Yes it's to do with your father's genes, isn't it, because her mum is 94. We assume that it's the father, there is a very very remote chance that it is her mother, but it looks like her father, but her father was clumsy, that's all.

For Sarah, one of the greatest losses associated with having HD was the surrender of her driving licence. Since Sarah and Max lived in a rural area, driving was a very important aspect of Sarah's life and using the car gave her independence and the ability to see friends and family and to do the shopping when she chose. Max expressed his view of how this had made Sarah feel:

Max: So really her whole world changed. It was like a guillotine coming down: 'I can't drive any more.' That was her whole life, going out, going everywhere. I was still at work.

Max continued to work for about 18 months after Sarah's diagnosis but it became apparent that Sarah could not be left on her own for long periods and he decided to take early retirement.

Max: Of course then she started falling down the stairs and things like that at home and the incontinence got worse and worse and it came to the point that she couldn't look after herself. I had to retire, so I did.

At the time of their first interview in November 2007, Sarah and Max were managing at home with just input from their HD specialist nurse, and the wider team from the outpatients' clinic. There are only a handful of specialist nurses for HD in the UK so this is a fairly unique and unusual service.

Max: But we were already with [a consultant neurologist], so [the HD specialist nurse] picked us up from that. And from being sort of out in the wilderness one month, the next month we had [the HD specialist nurse] to look after us, we had a dietician, we had a speech therapist, we had a consultant, and everything, and we had this team wrapped around us. And then I got involved with the Huntington's Disease Association, so there was a secondary form of support and everything. And from being very lost, lonely and bewildered, the structure is out there for you to become part of a group if you like. The feeling of isolation goes, there's people there you can get in contact with and everything, which of course I'm now part of. And without that, it would have been a pretty horrid time.

Max explains how the team helped with the different aspects of care:

> *Max:* We go to [clinic], I mean I don't count, if I have got a problem and say 'Look I need to come to a clinic quickly because we have got a problem', then [the HD specialist nurse] fits me in. I don't know, once every 6 months or so. . . . But in the meantime, they have been worried about Sarah's weight and things like that so [the dietician] comes out to see us. They were worried about Sarah's chewing the last visit so there is no food [at the clinic] to see it, . . . so [the speech and language therapist] arranged to come [to the house]. And [the HD specialist nurse] comes [to the house].

In the last couple of years Sarah's health has been deteriorating and she is no longer able to walk safely. Her 24 hour care became too much for Max on his own, despite respite periods throughout the year. The local social services arranged a package of care for Sarah to help alleviate the physical and emotional work for Max.

> *Max:* I now have a package of help from the local authority. And they come in the morning to get her up, just one girl comes in the mornings, it's easy in the mornings. And then at night, two girls come in to shower her and everything.

Max used to have an active social life and was able to follow a number of interests. He was also able to go to local support group meetings in the evening. However, Sarah could not be left in case she fell while on her own:

> *Max:* The biggest blow to Sarah was losing her independence. And I guess that impacted on me because I suddenly had to find a night to go out [food] shopping. . . . I started to go the carers group, those were evening meetings. And I could put her to bed and I was fairly confident that she'd be alright. Now I daren't do it, I daren't leave her by herself. So all my sort of . . . well there is virtually no evening activity at all, I just never ever go out.

The package of care worked well until Max had a mild stroke while Sarah was in respite care in late 2007. Luckily the care facility where Sarah was having respite was able to continue to care for her and it has now been decided that it is not possible for her to go home:

> *Max:* And then it became obvious that I couldn't look after her, not only from a physical sense, I mean I'm still a little bit un[steady] although I'm far better than I was. And they said 'Look, you've had all the stress and everything for five years, if you ever felt you were able to look after her once more it's going to happen again [risk of another stroke].' So we made a decision just after Christmas that she would have to stay there.

A case was put together for funding and, after initially being turned down, an appeal resulted in a fully funded place at a specialist care home for Sarah.

> *Max:* If they hadn't funded Sarah, then we'd have had a major problem, because our . . . expenditure would have exceeded our income by a vast amount.

Max visits her regularly and Sarah is getting on well with the staff and enjoys going out whenever she can:

> *Max:* They go to Birmingham to the Science Museum, they go to Manchester, they go to Sheffield. And there's only room for four on the bus, and she gets miffed, especially when it's football because all the men go to football. And the fact that she doesn't like football doesn't matter, it's the fact that she's going out and that's what she used to like to do. And so her coat is always with her, she won't leave her coat upstairs, it's always downstairs, her anorak, it's always round the back of her wheel-chair because if there's a seat on the bus she's there with her coat on saying I want to go out. So I mean I think she's . . . well in fact I'm very pleased at the way she's settled down, because it could have gone the other way.

Sarah seems to understand that she now lives at the care home and no longer asks when she can go home when her husband comes to visit. Max is recovering well from his stroke and physiotherapy has improved his walking, but he finds it very lonely at home by himself:

> *Max:* [It's] strange. Learning to live by yourself . . . there's two sides to it. There's the sort of physical side of it, there's nobody there, there's nobody for hugs and kisses when you need them, and I'm sure she needs them as much as I do, and just having someone to talk to, even if there's some-body there to listen as it were. There was a purpose if you like, I mean

I was looking after Sarah, that was my role, and I thought that we were doing very, very well – I didn't feel under stress. Now having said that, both the social workers and [the HD specialist nurse] were not surprised, and they'd all said make sure you keep going to the doctor, make sure you're all right. And I'm saying 'Yeah, yeah, I'm all right, you're fussing about nothing.'

Max is still very much involved in Sarah's care and visits her several times a week to spend time with her and take her out. At her last clinic appointment, the HD team were pleased with her condition and it was felt her speech showed some improvement.

Sarah and Max's experience illustrates some of the challenges of living with HD, not only for the person with the condition, but also their family carers and the health and social care professionals supporting their care needs. Their story demonstrates how situations can change, sometimes rapidly, requiring responsive care provision. In these circumstances helping the person with HD and their family to adapt to new challenges can be a significant part of a professional's role.

A NOTE ABOUT CHALLENGES IN RESEARCH WITH PEOPLE AFFECTED BY PLTNCs

Qualitative research that seeks to explore the experiences of those affected by PLTNCs is limited. This patient group presents particular challenges for researchers, which must be acknowledged. Cognitive impairments and communication difficulties present challenges for researchers in terms of complex ethical issues during recruitment and data collection. However, with the support and help of people with considerable experience in caring in their arena, adapted information sheets and consent forms to allow for reading, memory and physical deficits, and additional time and effort, people with PLTNCs need not be excluded from research and family caregivers need not be solely used as proxies for eliciting information.

Data collection periods during research with people with PLTNCs need to be flexible and not tied by a rigid time scale. Any data collection is dependent on participants' ability and willingness to spend their time with you. For example, on a visit to see how Sarah was settling into the residential care home, she did not wish to talk and it was not possible to conduct the interview; however, when next seen at a clinic visit she was happy to talk and for a researcher to accompany her to see the health professionals during her appointment. Those with PLTNCs have complex and often finely balanced lives; understanding and adaptability is a critical to the success of any research in the field.

Cognitive deficits can require a researcher to adapt their interview technique.

For example, people with PLTNCs can take longer to process and therefore need a little longer to respond to questions. People with HD can also find it difficult to process more than one question or complex information, requiring questions to use simple language and to only focus on one element at a time. Broad open ended questions may be too open and can often elicit a question in return or a one word answer. More direct questions or giving options to select from can sometimes be more useful. Speech impairments can present practical problems in that speech may be slurred, very quiet or shouting. Each of these aspects can make audio recordings difficult to transcribe and understand.

Due to the longevity and nature of PLTNCs it is not feasible or desirable for a person to be under constant supervision from any health or social care professional. The majority of their long-term care will be provided by family caregivers. Thus it is essential to improve our understanding of all aspects of living with these diseases by engaging with the real experts, people with PLTNCs and their informal care and support networks. Being aware of the complexity of the disease and challenges it may present for research is essential to optimise data collection and minimise negative effects for participants.

CONCLUSION

This chapter has focused on the impact of PLTNCs on patients and their families and draws together some of the key issues for care raised by these conditions. A case study from ongoing work has been utilised to illustrate some of these issues in a live context.

Provision of care for people with these conditions is predominantly provided by family/informal carers in the domestic home. Hence supporting this vital caring resource is essential. People with PLTNCs can experience cognitive and physical decline over extensive periods of time, requiring increasing input from family and professional carers. For families, care roles include physical and emotional aspects as well as the need to cope with losing the contributions of the person with the condition to aspects of family life such as income, household chores and raising children.

Care provided by health professionals needs to be timely and flexible in order to meet the differing and changing needs of patients. A multidisciplinary approach is advocated, but this requires coordination and good communication, often making a 'key worker' role essential for families to successfully navigate care systems. Due to the long-term nature of PLTNCs, attempts to incorporate self management and self referral have shown promise in a small number of studies and warrant further exploration.

Lastly the chapter points to some of the challenges of conducting research in this field and recommends the adaptation of standard research techniques in order to appropriately access and engage people with PLTNCs and their families.

A scarcity of literature in this field requires us to continue to make efforts to find ways to draw on the expertise of those affected by these conditions to create an evidence base to contribute to future provision of services.

REFERENCES

1 Department of Health. *The National Service Framework for Long-term (Neurological) Conditions.* London: COI; 2005.

2 Department of Health. *White Paper: Our Health, Our Care, Our Say: a new direction for community services.* London: COI; 2006.

3 Kelly M, Cats M. Hospice care in motor neurone disease. *Nurs Stand.* 1994; 9(9): 30–2.

4 O'Brien T, Kelly M, Saunders, C. Motor neurone disease: a hospice perspective. *BMJ.* 1992; **304**(6825): 471–3.

5 Oliver D. Palliative care for motor neurone disease. *Pract Neurol.* 2002; 2(2): 68–79.

6 Oliver D. The quality of care and symptom control: effects on the terminal phase of ALS/MND. *J Neurol Sci.* 1996; **139**(Suppl.): S134–6.

7 Oliver D, Webb S. The involvement of specialist palliative care in the care of people with motor neurone disease. *Palliat Med.* 2000; 14: 427–8.

8 Skelton J. Caring for patients with motor neurone disease. *Nurs Stand.* 1996; **10**(32): 33–6.

9 Skelton J. Nursing role in the multidisciplinary management of motor neurone disease. *Br J Nurs.* 2005; **14**(1): 20–4.

10 Wilson E, Elkan R, Seymour J, et al. A UK literature review of progressive long-term neurological conditions. *Br J Community Nurs.* 2008; **13**(5): 206–12.

11 Lee M, Walker R, Prentice W. The role of palliative care in Parkinson's disease. *Geriatric Medicine.* 2004; **34**(4): 51–4.

12 Thomas S, MacMahon D. *Parkinson's disease, palliative care and older people: Part 1. Nursing Older People.* 2004; **16**(1): 22–6.

13 Edmonds P, Vivat B, Burman R, et al. Loss and change: experiences of people severely affected by multiple sclerosis. *Palliat Med.* 2007; 21: 101–7.

14 Bourne C, Clayton C, Murch A, et al. Cognitive impairment and behavioural difficulties in patients with Huntington's disease. *Nurs Stand.* 2006; **20**(35): 41–4.

15 Kirkwood SC, Su JL, Conneally P, et al. Progression of symptoms in the early and middle stages of Huntington disease. *Arch Neurol.* 2001; **58**(2): 273–8.

16 Wade DT, Gage H, Owen C, et al. Multidisciplinary rehabilitation for people with Parkinson's disease: a randomised controlled study. *J Neurol Neurosurg Psychiatr.* 2003; **74**(2): 158–62.

17 Goldstein L, Adamson M, Jeffrey L, et al. The psychological impact of MND on patients and carers. *J Neurol Sci.* 1998; **160**(Suppl. 1): S114–21.

18 Brown J. User, carer and professional experiences of care in motor neurone disease. *Primary Health Care Research and Development.* 2003; 4: 207–17.

19 Carter J, Stewart B, Archbold P, et al. Living with a person who has Parkinson's disease: the spouse's perspective by stage of disease. *Move Disord.* 1998; **13**(1): 20–8.

20 Ray RA, Street AF. Caregiver bodywork: family members' experiences of caring for a person with motor neurone disease. *J Adv Nurs.* 2006; **56**(1): 35–43.

21 Tyler A, Harper PS, Davies K, *et al.* Family break-down and stress in Huntington's chorea. *J Biosoc Sci.* 1983; **15**: 127–38.

22 Kessler S. Forgotten person in the Huntington's disease family. *Am J Med Genet (Neuropsychiatric Genetics).* 1993; **48**: 145–50.

23 Twigg J, Atkin K. *Carers Perceived.* Buckingham: Open University Press; 1994.

24 Pollard J. *A Caregiver's Handbook for Advanced-Stage Huntington's Disease.* Ontario: Huntington's Disease Society of Canada; 1999.

25 Paulsen J. *Understanding Behaviour in Huntington's Disease: a practical guide for individuals, families, and professionals coping with HD.* Ontario: Huntington's Disease Society of Canada; 1999.

26 Semple O. The experiences of family members of persons with Huntington's disease. *Perspectives.* 1995; **19**(4): 4–10.

27 van Teijlingen E, Friend E, Kamal A. Service use and needs of people with motor neurone disease and their carers in Scotland. *Health Soc Care Community.* 2001; **9**(6): 396–403.

28 Aubeeluck A, Buchanan H. Capturing the Huntington's disease spousal carer experience. *Dementia.* 2006; **5**(1): 95–116.

29 Nolan M. Positive aspects of caring. In: Payne S, Ellis-Hill C, editors. *Chronic and Terminal Illness: new perspectives on caring and carers.* Oxford: Oxford University Press; 2001. pp. 22–43.

30 McGarva K. Huntington's disease: seldom seen – seldom heard? *Health Bull (Edinb).* 2001; **59**(5): 306–8.

31 O'Hara L, Cadbury H, De Souza L, *et al.* Evaluation of the effectiveness of professionally guided self care for people with multiple sclerosis living in the community: a randomized controlled trial. *Clin Rehabil.* 2002; **16**: 119–28.

32 Castleton B, Dunstan C, Nicholas V, *et al.* Improving care for patients with Parkinson's disease. *British Journal of Health Care Management.* 2005; **11**(4): 111–14.

33 MacLurg K, Reilly P, Hawkins S, *et al.* A primary care-based need assessment of people with multiple sclerosis. *Br J Gen Pract.* 2005; **55**(514): 378–83.

34 Trend P, Kaye J, Gage H, *et al.* Short-term effectiveness of intensive multidisciplinary rehabilitation for people with Parkinson's disease and their carers. *Clin Rehabil.* 2002; **16**: 717–25.

35 Hughes R, Aspinal F, Higginson I, *et al.* Assessing palliative care outcomes for people with motor neurone disease living at home. *Int J Palliat Nurs.* 2004; **10**(9): 449–53.

36 Holloway M. Traversing the network: a user-led care pathway approach to the management of Parkinson's disease in the community. *Health Soc Care Community.* 2005; **14**(1): 63–7.

37 Makepeace R, Barnes M, Semlyen J, *et al.* The establishment of a community multiple sclerosis team. *Int J Rehabil Res.* 2001; **24**: 137–41.

38 Matherson F, Porter B. The evolution of a relapse clinic for multiple sclerosis: challenges and recommendations. *Br J Neurosci Nurs.* 2006; **2**(4): 180–6.

39 Lloyd M. Where has all the care management gone? The challenge of Parkinson's disease to the health and social care interface. *Br J Soc Work.* 2000; **30**: 737–54.

CHAPTER 7

Palliative initiatives in neurological care: the PINC programme

Judi Byrne and Pam McClinton

As previous chapters have discussed, the need for palliative care for a person with a progressive long-term neurological condition (PLTNC) is increasingly being recognised, particularly for those with a rapidly degenerative condition such as MND.[1] However, this recognition also highlights the challenges in providing services to this group of patients and the need for specialist palliative care services to provide care outside of the traditional cancer arena and the acute hospital care setting.

This chapter will critically consider some of these challenges to equitable community based care, and give an example of voluntary sector and NHS care providers coming together through the use of best practice tools to provide integrated neurological palliative care at the end of life.

INTRODUCTION

Historically, advances in end of life care have centred on people dying from cancer,[2] even though this equates to only 25% of the total number of deaths in the UK.[3] Therefore, until quite recently, the knowledge and skills of palliative care professionals have been focused on giving care to this particular group of adult cancer patients, based primarily in a hospice or hospital location with some community outreach.

It is predominantly specialist palliative care for cancer patients which the national charity Sue Ryder Care provides from its six hospices spread across England. However, the charity is unique in that it also offers specialist neurological care from seven centres covering England and Scotland. Because of this uniqueness the charity is well placed to highlight the challenges and potential solutions to providing equitable palliative care in both cancer and PLTNCs.

National policy increasingly reflects the broad trend which has moved from a narrow focus on the needs of people with cancer to a focus on the needs of a wider group of the population, including those with neurological conditions, who have palliative care needs in the last years or months of life. The need for palliative care in neurological conditions, including the potential input from specialist palliative care professionals, has been highlighted in various policy initiatives. Chief among these is the Department of Health National End of Life Care Strategy,[4] advocating improved end of life care for all patients regardless of diagnosis. Additional impetus has come from, for example, the National Institute for Health and Clinical Excellence (NICE) guidance on multiple sclerosis, or Parkinson's disease.[5,6] The National Service Framework for Long-term (Neurological) Conditions has made recommendations for the provision of palliative care services to support people with neurological conditions throughout and to the end of their lives. It does this in the context of its 11 Quality Requirements (QRs).[7]

Staff who work within neurological centres in Sue Ryder Care caring for people with PLTNCs experience at first hand the difficulties and barriers to accessing optimum palliative care recommended in national policy. These are summarised in Box 7.1.

BOX 7.1 Challenges for palliative care for PLTNCs

- Being able to identify when people are coming to the end of life stage. Frequently people die a sudden 'unexpected' death and in these circumstances the opportunity to move towards and provide palliative care is missed.
- Many people have multifaceted disabilities which include communication limitations, and cognitive and behavioural problems, as well as complex physical disability.
- Staff are experienced in caring for people who cannot communicate verbally with them and other health and social professionals may find it challenging to manage someone with profound cognitive dysfunction.
- Everyday skills used for postural management and physical handling, e.g. for someone with severe spasticity, are common in the care centres, but these elements of care are seen infrequently in palliative care literatures.

Much of the palliative care research evidence used is drawn from expertise gained in relation to cancer, although more recently there has been increased interest in broadening knowledge and skills to a wider range of different diagnoses, particularly chronic disease, at the end of life.

GENERALIST PALLIATIVE CARE PROVISION

A model for provision of palliative care is that it should be provided by generalists and specialists working together across geographical locations and professional boundaries.[8] It is a model which proposes generalist palliative care being provided by general practitioners (GPs) and district nurses (DNs) and specialist palliative care by clinical nurse specialists and palliative care consultants, working in hospitals and hospices, with some having a joint community provision remit, for the most part to cancer patients.

Evidence from the Primary Care Neurological Society is that a number of GPs either lack the skills or the confidence to manage people presenting with neurological symptoms.[10] Other research indicates that neurological care is sometimes patchy, overstretched and insensitive to individual patients' needs.[9] It has also been found that communication between the patient and the health professional and between different sectors of the health service is sometimes poor and may lead to time wasting and delays in treatment.[9] Patients and their carers responding to a postal survey by the United Brain Tumour Campaign expressed doubts about a GP's knowledge or awareness of the complexities of managing neurological conditions and reported that they were less satisfied with the service from their GP than hospital.[11] In conjunction with this a survey by the Parkinson's Disease Society (PDS) found that one in five GPs did not refer people with suspected PD to a specialist and one in four changed medication without referral.[12] The PDS reported that although GPs may have as many as three or four people with PD in their caseload, up to 96% admit to having no specialist knowledge of the condition.[12]

Community teams could therefore benefit from further training not only in palliative care but also to support them in caring for people with severe motor, sensory, cognitive and/or communication impairments as a result of a neurological condition.[13] In the community, families and social care staff give day to day care with the GP and DN providing medical and nursing care as a backup to this mainstay. A small number of centres in the UK offer specialised care for people in the advanced stages of neurological conditions, and the charity organisation Sue Ryder Care is one of the main providers.

SPECIALIST PALLIATIVE CARE PROVISION

The remit of specialist palliative care services extends from acute hospital care through to provision in the community and hospice care which is principally provided by the charitable sector.

Traditional hospice based care has been mostly associated with caring for people with advanced cancer, and hospices may be less experienced in caring for people with other conditions. One of the differences between the cancer trajectory and that associated with neurological conditions is that the latter may involve a protracted course of illness with people needing palliatively focused care over an extended period of time to alleviate symptoms and improve their quality of life. Yet many symptoms experienced by cancer patients and people with neurological conditions are similar: cancer patients' symptoms may be more severe, but those of non cancer patients tend to be more prolonged.[13] These prolonged symptoms are varied, and many people have complex disabilities which include a mix of communication, behavioural and cognitive problems as well as physical limitations.[14]

The cancer focus of most existing palliative care services, together with the difficulties of recognising when patients with neurological conditions are entering the end of life period, has meant that people living in the community with neurological conditions and at the end of their lives may not have their palliative and end of life care needs adequately assessed or met. This situation is particularly challenging in other care settings outside of the NHS, and is partly due to a lack of access to a wider range of specialist services but also to a lack of knowledge and skills among care professionals on how to provide neurological palliative care. Despite some advances in raising awareness, research shows that only a small proportion of people with non cancer related palliative care needs can access the services.[15]

GOOD PRACTICE EXAMPLE OF IMPROVING PALLIATIVE CARE IN NEUROLOGICAL CARE SETTINGS

The Sue Ryder Care Palliative Initiatives in Neurological Care programme (PINC) joined together the charity's expertise as a provider of long-term neurological care and its specialist palliative care hospice services to address an inequality of care provision and open up the choices at the end of life for people with neurological conditions living in its neurological care centres.

The specialised neurological care centres provide full time nursing care for residents with a wide range of sudden onset and intermittent PLTNCs. As with the general population, those living in the neurological care centres access other healthcare needs via their GP, including referral and access to specialist palliative care teams. Historically specialist palliative care teams have only become involved for people with a diagnosis of cancer and issues of criteria and referral processes for people with PLTNCs have been anecdotally cited.

The Sue Ryder Care hospices care for patients on a needs rather than diagnosis basis, however the majority of patients do have a cancer diagnosis. The hospice team is led by palliative care consultants with some services extending into the community.

THE PALLIATIVE INITIATIVES IN NEUROLOGICAL CARE (PINC) PROGRAMME

Through the specialised neurological care centres, and supported by the Sue Ryder Care hospices, PINC adapted and piloted the nationally recognised best practice care tools: Gold Standards Framework in Care Homes (GSFCH); Liverpool Care Pathway for the Dying Patient (LCP); and Preferred Priorities of Care (PPC) to evaluate their potential to improve palliative care and end of life care for people with PLTNCs living in a nursing care environment.

The key drivers for this work were not only the increasing profile for neuro palliative care and end of life care nationally, but also organisational recognition that the palliative care needs of people who die in the care centres could be improved. This acknowledgement of need for improvement was focused on areas of staff difficulty in recognising or supporting impending death; lack of knowledge and implementation of best practice in the initial assessment of care; in anticipatory planning; communication; care after a death; and a limited knowledge of and access to palliative care resources.

PINC worked with the NHS End of Life Care Initiative to pilot best practice care tools within a neurological care setting. The NHS End of Life Care Initiative was launched in 2004 to improve end of life care for people, irrespective of diagnosis. It also sought to give people greater choice in their place of care and death. This included reducing the number of crisis admissions to acute care of those who had expressed a wish to die at the centre, as well as reducing the number of patients transferred from care homes to acute care in the last weeks of life.[16]

Key to achieving these aims was the dissemination of the three care tools, which were endorsed by the National Institute for Health and Clinical Excellence in 2004. These are GSFCH, LCP, and PPC (now Preferred Priorities *for* Care).[16]

BEST PRACTICE TOOLS

The Gold Standards Framework in Care Homes (GSFCH) Tool

The GSFCH was developed and modified from the primary care sectors who implement the Gold Standards Framework (GSF) model to optimise the organisation, communication and proactive planning for people in the last years of life living in care homes.

The tool focuses particularly on improving the collaboration with primary care and the GPs who look after patients in care homes. Based on the principles of the GSF to 'identify, assess and plan care' and using key tasks, templates and assessment tools, the GSFCH supports palliative care in the care home and enables integrated collaborative working with primary care and specialist teams.

GSFCH processes are to:

1 identify and raise awareness using a supportive care register, communication meetings and audit

2 assess needs both physical and psychosocial, and use validated assessment tools

3 plan ahead for problems, including preference for place of care, GP and out of hours support, and resident and family support.[16]

The Liverpool Care Pathway for the Dying Patient (LCP) Tool

The LCP[18] was developed to take the hospice care model into caring for people in hospital and other settings including care homes. It is used to care for patients in the last days or hours of life once it is recognised that they are dying. The LCP involves promoting good communication with the patient and family, anticipatory planning including psychosocial and spiritual needs, symptom control (pain, agitation, and respiratory tract secretions) and care after death. The LCP has accompanying symptom control guidelines and information leaflets for relatives.

It consists of three sections.

Section 1: Baseline assessment

This section acknowledges and opens the discussions about the fact that the patient is dying. It promotes honest, sensitive, timely discussions, a proactive approach to symptom management and recognition of the importance of psychological, spiritual, religious, cultural and family needs. Although the patient and family may well have been assessed previously, the reality of facing the dying process can significantly impact on previously expressed beliefs and wishes and the need for information.

Section 2: Ongoing assessment

This section provides the prompts and goals of patient care that need to be assessed and monitored frequently to ensure that the patient's comfort is maintained and that the patient as well as the family is supported throughout the dying process. In an inpatient environment goals are assessed and documented at least 4 hourly. If goals are not met they are recorded as a variance with the reason for this clearly stated as well as the action taken to resolve meeting the goal.

Section 3: Care after death

This section is completed after the patient has died. The main drive of the goals is to ensure that the patient has received appropriate care and that the family are supported, know what to do following the death and are given access to bereavement literature.[17]

Preferred Priorities for Care (PPC) Tool

The PPC[19] provides a mechanism to record patients' and carers' preferences, audit patient experiences, monitor patients' trajectory of care during the palliative stage of a disease, and also highlights variance from the preferred care plan.

The PPC is a document that the patient creates and takes with them as they receive care in different places. It has space for the patients' thoughts about their care and the choices they would like to make, including saying where they would want to be when they die. If anything changes, this is written in the plan so it remains up to date.[18]

PINC PROGRAMME AIMS

PINC aimed to develop and pilot these tools, improve processes and communication structures and deliver palliative care education packages across the centres to meet the complex care needs of people with PLTNCs at the end of life.

The project involved 238 residents ranging in age from 20 years to over 85 years, and over 300 nursing and care staff in six care centres around England where PINC worked to coordinate local links with health and social care providers to improve care.

OUTCOMES

Overall, project evaluation has suggested that PINC has had an impact on several levels. It has sparked a renewed interest from staff in palliative and end of life care, promoted the development and documentation of practice and kindled enthusiasm for further training and education in a wide range of palliative and end of life care areas.

The pilot has enabled staff to learn how palliative care for a non malignant diagnosis differs from that of cancer and what these differences mean to delivery of every day care and use of finite resources.

There have been increased opportunities to work in partnership with other organisations both in the voluntary sector and the NHS. The sharing of resources, and delivery of palliative and end of life care training modules has been utilised to minimise costs for everyone.

THE TOOLS

> 'Yes, and I like having the tools in place, so I know what I'm doing. There's a guideline, something that I can do, and I'm not sort of panicking and thinking oh my god, what am I going to do?'
>
> (Care centre staff focus group response)

Gold Standards Framework in Care Homes (GSFCH)

The pilot has demonstrated that the adapted GSFCH tool can be an effective and appropriate tool to facilitate best practice for quality end of life care in neurological care centres. Four of the pilot centres developed active supportive care registers with needs banding for all residents. The register considered their palliative care status, anticipated needs and health team input, along with individual supportive care sheets to aid communication with out of hours (OOH) providers and ambulance crews.

The learning from this was:

➤ prognostication for residents is more guess work than science. Those with a possible year to live (A) can die suddenly, those with perceived days (D) can be recoded back up again as they improve
➤ processes are only as good as the communication links they use. Strong links with GPs and OOH providers are key.

Liverpool Care Pathway for the Dying Patient (LCP)

The LCP was the most difficult to adapt because its clinical focus made it challenging to use in these care settings without in house medical cover. However, use of the LCP in three care centres has facilitated greater openness around dying, with nurses becoming more proactively aware of residents' changing needs as death approaches. The LCP has been significantly adapted to suit people with PLTNCs, and could be appropriate for use with patients with dementia.

As a result:

➤ nursing practice can now focus on symptom control and comfort measures and is not as task orientated
➤ access to syringe drivers and medication when needed, generalist knowledge for neurological symptom control, prescribing, and specialist palliative input remain challenging but are being addressed by working with healthcare professionals locally.

Preferred Priorities for Care (PPC)

Use of the PPC has improved staff competency in advocating for residents and/ or their family, particularly in relation to their expressed views about their preferred place of care. Staff also report feeling more comfortable in talking about end of life care with residents. Over the course of the pilot, opportunities for conversations surrounding PPC increased in the three pilot centres, suggesting the tool served as a prompt to encourage discussion and communication about residents' choice. Ninety-nine per cent of residents recorded the care centres as their preferred place of care at end of life. The remaining 1% wished to return to the family home.

The results highlighted the following.

➤ Staff confidence has increased both in approaching residents and families and in challenging clinical decisions about place of care.
➤ Despite the cognitive impairments of the majority of residents, there are ways for those who know them well, such as the nursing staff, to communicate and find out their choices, but it takes time and perseverance.

THE CARE @ DEATH AUDIT TOOL

The number of residents who die is relatively small (the average is 19% per year across the six centres), nevertheless in recognition of the importance of having robust processes to capture evidence of the quality of care, a Care @ Death audit tool was developed. This audit tool has 27 questions to complete after a resident's death which are a mix of demographics, use of care tools, MDT input and a section for staff to reflect on what did and didn't go so well and their learning from the experience.

Through this audit, case studies and focus group work with staff and families, a picture is being built which more accurately reflects a neurological care of the dying pathway. As a result a PINC Pathway for Care at the End of Life aimed for use in care home settings and incorporating the three care tools has begun to evolve. This pathway could provide a standard service model for end of life care

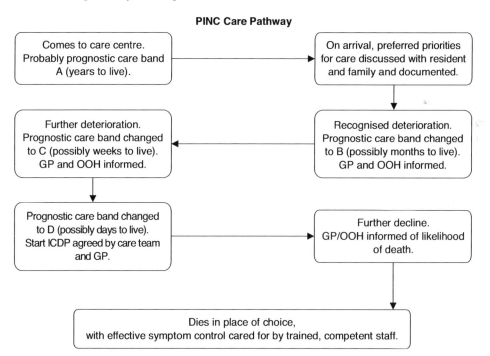

PINC Care Pathway

Comes to care centre. Probably prognostic care band A (years to live).	On arrival, preferred priorities for care discussed with resident and family and documented.
Further deterioration. Prognostic care band changed to C (possibly weeks to live). GP and OOH informed.	Recognised deterioration. Prognostic care band changed to B (possibly months to live). GP and OOH informed.
Prognostic care band changed to D (possibly days to live). Start ICDP agreed by care team and GP.	Further decline. GP/OOH informed of likelihood of death.

Dies in place of choice, with effective symptom control cared for by trained, competent staff.

FIGURE 7.1 PINC pathway for end of life care

which may result in identified service specifications and performance criteria that can be shared with commissioners (*see* Figure 7.1)

CHALLENGES TO CHANGE

At the start of the project, residents, their families and key local stakeholders were invited to project launch events. Invites were sent to a mix of GPs, DNs, specialist palliative care teams, cancer network staff, social workers and commissioners who all had a part to play in the care delivered at the centre. The events introduced PINC, opened up communication links and paved the way for collaborative working with stakeholders.

These events were followed up by the PINC programme lead and care centre link teams focusing on adapting and implementing the care tools and identifying specific areas for improvement (*see* Box 7.1).

BOX 7.2 Adapting and implementing the care tools in care centres

> For two centres this was their OOH provision. Working with the OOH provider and the sharing of information and processes has resulted in the adaptation of their local OOH database so that it now includes all residents at the centre, allowing on-call doctors to have access to detailed information about a residents' neurological condition before visiting.
>
> A care centre focus group member commented:
>
>> So they'll hopefully be more familiar with our client group, and the present state of their illness. So that's something that's coming up, a real positive.
>>
>> (Care centre focus group response)
>
> For another centre the working relationship with the GP and specialist palliative care team was identified as a block to improving care. Meetings were held where issues around support and access were discussed and resolved.
>
>> I think they've improved in that area, now we've got a line of communication with them. We have meetings with them. They're aware that we're doing PINC and they're fully supportive, aren't they, with what we're doing.
>>
>> (Care centre focus group response)

DEVELOPING WORKFORCE SKILLS AND KNOWLEDGE

Initially, PINC related education was viewed as being mainly concerned with the piloting of the tools and the changes in documentation. However, in the process of educating staff about implementing the end of life care tools, a lack of knowledge of the basic tenets of palliative care among some nursing and support staff became apparent. Staff feedback showed that care centre staff required basic and enhanced training in areas including general palliative care, communication skills, particularly for bereavement, and more focused disease specific training.

The PINC education and training needs assessment exercise identified a lack of basic palliative care knowledge for the majority of National Vocational Qualification (NVQ) level 2 and 3 support staff, along with varying levels of skills and knowledge among clinical nursing staff, quality and access to education and training resources, both internal and external to Sue Ryder Care.

To address these issues the PINC programme worked with each pilot centre to produce their Palliative Care Training Plan including the care toolkit; to implement the Macmillan Foundations in Palliative Care Programme for NVQ level 2 and 3 staff; and to source and negotiate for external education resources.

A pilot for Essentials in Neurological Palliative Care, an internal education programme for senior nurses, was run to build on palliative care knowledge. This pilot was developed in response to an identified lack of specialised neuro palliative care training resources.

> And the study days that we do, we then talk about cancer, talk about this happens and then that happens. It's a much more defined way of looking at palliative care and looking at end of life care. But here it's different.
>
> (Care centre focus group response)

The practice of registered nurses verifying expected deaths is now common practice in many hospitals and primary care trusts. With the emphasis on enhanced care at the end of life, it was helpful for Sue Ryder Care nurses, particularly for those working in residential settings, to be able to formally verify the expected deaths of a patient. A policy and comprehensive training package was developed for qualified nursing staff and the procedure has now been rolled out across both hospice and neurological care centres.

CONCLUSION

➤ With the adapted models Sue Ryder Care has found the end of life care tools can be used successfully for people with PLTNCs. The result of this is a PINC Pathway for End of Life Care, incorporating the adapted tools, for neurological care centre residents at end of life. This pathway can provide a standard service model for end of life care, which it is hoped will result in identified service specifications and performance criteria that can be shared with commissioners.

➤ Using this pathway, PINC has begun to integrate the knowledge, skills and experience of specialist palliative care, with that of neurology professionals, to provide the same comprehensive approach to neurological palliation at the end of life as has evolved in specialist care for cancer.

➤ Keys to success are strong links with local healthcare providers who work in partnership with committed, palliative care trained staff to deliver proactive, evidenced based care at the end of life.

Overall, project evaluation has suggested that the PINC programme has had an impact on several levels. It has sparked a renewed interest from staff in palliative and end of life care, promoted the development and documentation of practice and kindled enthusiasm for further training and education in a wide range of palliative and end of life care areas.

The programme has enabled staff to learn how palliative care for a non malignant diagnosis differs from that of cancer, and what these differences mean to delivery of care and use of resources.

It is hoped that other care providers can use these findings to support the delivery of neurological end of life care as an acknowledged part of healthcare service provision. PINC will continue to work to demonstrate how the best possible use is being made of limited resources to ensure that people continue to be supported to die with dignity, free of pain, and in the setting of their choice regardless of the diagnosis.

REFERENCES

1 O'Brien T, Kelly M, Saunders C. Motor neurone disease: a hospice perspective. *BMJ.* 1992; **304**: 471–3.

2 Traue DC, Ross JR. Palliative care in non malignant disease. *J R Soc Med.* 2005; **98**: 503–6.

3 Cancer Research UK. *Cancer Key Facts.* London: Cancer Research UK; 2008.

4 Department of Health. *End of Life Care Strategy: promoting high quality care for all adults at the end of life.* London: DH; 2008.

5 National Institute for Health and Clinical Excellence. *Management of Multiple Sclerosis in Primary and Secondary Care: NICE guideline 8.* London: NICE; 2003. www.nice.org. uk/Guidance/CG8

6 National Institute for Health and Clinical Excellence. *Parkinson's Disease: diagnosis and management in primary and secondary care: NICE guideline 35.* London: NICE; 2006. www.nice.org.uk/Guidance/CG35

7 Department of Health. *The National Service Framework for Long-term (Neurological) Conditions.* London: COI; 2005.

8 Department of Health. *Our Health, Our Care, Our Say: a new direction for community services.* London: COI; 2006.

9 Smithson WH, Hukins D, Jones L. How general practice can help improve care of people with neurological conditions: a qualitative study. *Primary Health Care Research & Development.* 2006; **7**: 201–10.

10 Primary Care Neurological Society. *The P-CNS Business Plan.* London: P-CNS; 2006. Available at: www.p-cns.org.uk/PCNSBDP.pdf

11 United Brain Tumour Campaign. Survey of patients and carers affected by brain tumours. 2005. Available at: www.elliestrust.org/files/survey%20report%202005. doc

12 Parkinson's Disease Society. www.Parkinsons.org.uk

13 O'Brien A, Welsh J, Dunn FG. Clinical review ABC of palliative care: non-malignant conditions. *BMJ.* 1998; **316**: 286–9.

14 Royal College of Physicians, National Council for Palliative Care, British Society of Rehabilitation Medicine. *Long-term Neurological Conditions: management at the interface between neurology, rehabilitation and palliative care. Concise Guidance to Good Practice Series, No 10.* London: RCP; 2008.

15 Department of Health. *National Service Framework for Long-term (Neurological) Conditions.* op. cit.

16 End of Life Care for Adults Programme. www.endoflifecareforadults.nhs.uk/eolc

17 National Gold Standards Framework. www.goldstandardsframework.nhs.uk

18 Liverpool Care Pathway. www.mcpcil.org.uk/liverpool_care_pathway

19 Lancashire and South Cumbria Cancer Network. www.cancerlancashire.org.uk/ppc. html

Ethical considerations in the palliative care of patients with neurological disorders

Richard Partridge and Penny McNamara

INTRODUCTION

Difficult decisions in medical care need to be confronted and responded to in all aspects of practice. Medical advances at both ends of life, before birth and in prolonging life, seem to have blurred the distinction of where we consider life to start and end. Medical ethics concerns itself with the decision making in such difficult areas. The subject covers a vast range of aspects of medical care and incorporates philosophy, the law and moral codes. Caring for patients with neurological disorders can present numerous ethical challenges, right from diagnosis up to the latter stages of the illness. For instance, the diagnosis of these conditions often takes months to reach from the onset of symptoms, as previously discussed. During the investigative process the clinician is obliged to keep the patient appropriately informed, but may be reluctant to disclose all possible outcomes in order to minimise patient anxiety and distress. After diagnosis, the course of the illness may be unpredictable and the amount of information each patient desires should be sensitively explored. The patient will have to face the prospect of progressive loss of function, possible swallowing problems leading to feeding difficulties, respiratory problems and increasing difficulty communicating. These clinical problems create the ethical dilemmas of artificial feeding and ventilatory support. The loss of independence may lead some patients to question their quality of life and consider the futility of prolonging their existence. Some may also develop cognitive problems impairing capacity. The threat to capacity may raise issues of advance care planning or proxy decision making.

A good knowledge of these challenges and the ethical and legal issues that arise from them are essential for health professionals caring for such patients. Skilled communication and teamwork is essential and underpins all of this.

In this chapter we will give an overview of the relevant issues. We will start by outlining an ethical framework for decision making and then summarise relevant legal considerations, in particular the general principles when considering treatment decisions including assessing capacity and the basic principles of the Mental Capacity Act 2005 (MCA). We will also include relevant case histories to illustrate some of the important points. What follows is necessarily brief and cannot hope to cover all the relevant issues but is intended more to give a flavour of some of the pertinent issues and how to approach them. For specific legal questions professional bodies and indemnity organisations may be helpful.

ETHICAL FRAMEWORKS

There are various ethical theories and ways of approaching ethical problems but 'principilism' as described by Beauchamp and Childress[1] has become a widely used ethical framework for considering moral dilemmas in medicine. It describes four clusters of moral principles that serve as a guideline for working through an ethical dilemma (*see* Box 8.1).

BOX 8.1 The four clusters of principilism

Respect for autonomy (patient choice)

In this context, autonomy has come to mean self rule or self determination. And respect for autonomy means that we should respect the right of patients to make their own choices about what happens to them. For instance, people should be able to choose what medical treatments they do or don't receive.

Beneficence (do the most good)

In simple terms, the duty to 'do good'. As health professionals we should aim to do good or what is best for our patients.

Non maleficence (do the least harm)

The duty to do no harm. To all intents and purposes beneficence and non maleficence can be seen as two sides of the same coin and one can't really be considered without the other. For instance, when considering a medical treatment's merit one must weigh the 'good' it will achieve with the potential harm.

Justice (fair allocation of resources)

Fairness to all; the duty to provide a fair distribution of resources.

These principles may appear quite straightforward when read in this way. However, their application in real life situations can be complex and challenging, especially where there is significant conflict between two or more of the principles. Great importance is placed on individual autonomy in our society. Respect for autonomy is fundamental to maintaining trust between doctor and patient and provides the benchmark for informed consent to treatment. In fact, a patient's right to decline treatment offered is protected by the law relating to consent. For instance, no one would argue against a competent cancer patient's right to decide whether or not to receive chemotherapy. The situation regarding treatment requests is more complex. A person should expect to be offered the best available treatments and the medical team should be expected to provide them. However, should the patient's autonomy be so absolute as to be able to demand whatever treatment they see fit, even if the treatment is considered to offer no benefit by the doctor? Rather, the doctor anticipates considerable burden to the patient. Let us consider the cancer patient again; should they be able to demand a chemotherapy treatment that has no chance of helping them but every chance of harming them in their desperate hope for a cure? The doctor may feel that their duty to do no harm (non maleficence) overrides respect for the patient's autonomy in this situation. Likewise, there may be an argument that this would be an inappropriate use of resources. The resources used to attempt a treatment that will not benefit a patient would not be available for use to treat another patient. This would seem to go against the principle of justice. Some of these issues were highlighted in the case of *Burke v General Medical Council* (*see* Box 8.2). This is a complex area ethically and legally and where there is doubt legal advice should be sought. However, some general principles regarding medical treatment can be applied as detailed in the next section.

BOX 8.2 *Burke v General Medical Council* (GMC)

In 2004 Mr Oliver Leslie Burke, aged 45, went to the High Court to challenge the GMC guidance on withholding and withdrawing life-prolonging treatment,[2,3] citing that it was incompatible with the Human Rights Act. Mr Burke has a condition known as cerebellar ataxia which is a progressive degenerative disorder that follows a similar course to multiple sclerosis. It was anticipated that as his condition deteriorated he would lose the ability to swallow and would require artificial nutrition and hydration (ANH) in order to survive.

ANH is a term used to describe various methods of providing nutrition or hydration to people who can't take them by mouth, e.g. PEG, nasogastric tube, intravenous infusion, subcutaneous infusion. It is now established in common law that artificial nutrition and hydration (ANH) is considered as medical treatment.[4]

Mr Burke wanted ANH to be provided to him right through to the end stage of his illness. He was concerned that the GMC guidance gave doctors the power to withdraw this treatment at a time when he was no longer able to communicate his wishes on the basis that they judged his life was no longer worth living – even if his death was not imminent. Medical evidence submitted to the court suggested that Mr Burke would likely retain capacity to make decisions about treatment until very near to his death.

In July 2004 Mr Justice Munby ruled in favour of Mr Burke and declared that parts of the guidance were incompatible with the Human Rights Act. This judgment was, however, overturned by the Court of Appeal in August 2005.[5] The Court of Appeal decided that the GMC guidance was lawful as it stood at the time. In particular, they felt that Mr Burke's concern that ANH could be stopped at a time when his death was not imminent was unfounded. They said that where a competent patient requests ANH that will be life prolonging then it must be provided and that there is nothing in the guidance to suggest otherwise. Moreover, they stated:

> Indeed, it seems to us that for a doctor deliberately to interrupt life-prolonging treatment in the face of a competent patient's expressed wish to be kept alive, with the intention of thereby terminating the patient's life, would leave the doctor with no answer to the charge of murder.[6]

However, they were quick to point out that this does not mean that a patient can demand whatever treatment they want but that there is a primary duty of care to take reasonable measures to keep a patient alive where this is their known wish. They further clarified this point:

> Autonomy and the right of self-determination do not entitle the patient to insist on receiving a particular medical treatment regardless of the nature of the treatment. Insofar as a doctor has a legal obligation to provide treatment this cannot be founded simply upon the fact that the patient demands it. The source of the duty lies elsewhere.[7]

A medical team, they note, has a positive duty of care for a patient that includes a duty to take such steps as are reasonable to keep the patient alive: 'Where ANH is necessary to keep the patient alive, the duty of care will normally require the doctors to supply ANH.'[8]

And further: 'Where the competent patient makes it plain that he or she wishes to be kept alive by ANH, this will not be the source of the duty to provide it. The patient's wish will merely underscore that duty.'[8]

It is important to note, however, that the duty to provide such treatment is only valid if the treatment is clinically indicated. In other words, a patient cannot demand a treatment (even ANH) if it is not clinically indicated. The Court of Appeal endorsed the following points put forward by the GMC:

> The doctor, exercising his professional clinical judgment, decides what treatment options are clinically indicated (i.e. will provide overall clinical benefit) for his patient.

He then offers those treatment options to the patient in the course of which he explains to him/her the risks, benefits, side effects, etc involved in each of the treatment options.

The patient then decides whether he wishes to accept any of those treatment options and, if so, which one. In the vast majority of cases he will, of course, decide which treatment option he considers to be in his best interests and, in doing so, he will or may take into account other, non clinical, factors. However, he can, if he wishes, decide to accept (or refuse) the treatment option on the basis of reasons which are irrational or for no reasons at all. If he chooses one of the treatment options offered to him, the doctor will then proceed to provide it.

If, however, he refuses all of the treatment options offered to him and instead informs the doctor that he wants a form of treatment which the doctor has not offered him, the doctor will, no doubt, discuss that form of treatment with him (assuming that it is a form of treatment known to him) but if the doctor concludes that this treatment is not clinically indicated he is not required (i.e. he is under no legal obligation) to provide it to the patient although he should offer to arrange a second opinion.[9]

GENERAL PRINCIPLES REGARDING MEDICAL TREATMENT

In addition to the ethical framework outlined above, it is imperative that healthcare practitioners act within the laws laid down by the society within which they practise. But it is worth noting that both moral norms and statute laws vary from one society to another. A good example of this variation in position is illustrated by therapeutic abortions. Within a society there may be variation in opinion, and the law governing such practice varies from country to country. An important piece of legislation to be considered in context of ethical issues for people with progressive long-term neurological conditions (PLTNCs) is the MCA.[10]

Medical treatments, whether trivial or life saving, should always be considered to be in the patient's best interests. For many hundreds of thousands of treatments that occur daily, the treatment is offered based on evaluating clinical information, evidence for the treatment and experience of the doctor. The treatment is offered to the patient and it is the collaboration of both parties and the resulting compliance that determines what is in the best interests for that individual. In these incidents the person receiving the treatment offer is able to exert his autonomy. While the doctor is obliged to offer only what he believes is in his patient's best interests, this may differ from the patient's view and the patient may refuse what is offered. The general principles for treatment decisions for patients with capacity and for patients without capacity are detailed in the next two sections.

For patients with capacity

In order to be autonomous and make their own informed choices about medical treatments, a patient must be competent to do so, i.e. have legal capacity and also be free from coercion. A patient is presumed to have capacity unless proven otherwise. The MCA outlines how to assess capacity (*see* p. 120 for further details).

➤ A patient with capacity must consent to treatment for it to be provided. They must also be provided with sufficient information to be able to reach a decision.

➤ A patient with capacity can decline medical treatment before or after it is started even if it is anticipated that this will cause harm to the patient or even lead to the patient's death.

➤ A patient with capacity cannot demand a treatment that a doctor believes is not in their best interests, i.e. that is medically futile or overly burdensome.[11]

For further, more detailed information see the GMC's guidance on consent to treatment.[11]

CASE EXAMPLE 8.1 Mr A

Mr A, aged 57, was diagnosed with motor neurone disease (MND) just six months ago but appears to have a rapidly progressive form of the illness. He cannot walk but can stand and transfer with the help of two people but will soon require hoisting. His speech has also deteriorated and is becoming markedly dysarthric. He has lost the ability to write and has not got on well with communication aids and had given up using these at present. He has recently started having some difficulty swallowing and has been losing weight. Mr A has been very reluctant to talk about his illness to date and appears frightened about what is happening to him. He previously didn't attend his appointment for consideration of percutaneous endoscopic gastrostomy (PEG) placement. Mr A's wife is very upset about his deterioration and feels that Mr A is being allowed to 'waste away'. She is putting a lot of pressure on the medical team to persuade Mr A to have a PEG to provide artificial nutrition and hydration (ANH).

What issues does the healthcare team need to consider in this situation?

• Does Mr A have capacity to decide about ANH?
• What discussions should take place with Mr A about his treatment options?
• What are the likely benefits and harms of receiving ANH in this context?

Mr A currently has capacity to make decisions about medical treatment and so the healthcare team should try to discuss with him his treatment options.

While Mrs A's concerns are understandable, the medical team should in no way try to 'persuade' Mr A to have a PEG. In order to be given the chance to make an informed autonomous choice about whether to receive ANH, he should be given the option to hear the relevant risks and benefits of proceeding with PEG placement, including what might happen in the future and how his care and symptoms could be managed with or without ANH. Mr A would also have the option to make an Advance Decision to Refuse Treatment (ADRT) or appoint a Lasting Power of Attorney (LPA). It is important to note, however, that his speech is rapidly deteriorating and every effort should be made to help him maximise his ability to communicate (i.e. through communication aids) but he will likely increasingly struggle to articulate his wishes as time goes by. It would be better to discuss such complex and sensitive advance care planning issues now while Mr A's communication is still at a level where this is possible. Skilled communication will be essential in talking to Mr A about his options. Clearly he is very frightened and a sensitive exploration of his thoughts and feelings about the situation is vital. Equally, Mr A should not be forced to talk about things that he does not want to.

For people with MND the placement of a PEG tube and provision of ANH may be life prolonging and may be associated with improved symptom control. Recent evidence has suggested that early placement produces better results (i.e. before swallowing and nutritional compromise sets in) and safer (before respiratory function deteriorates).[12] For some patients, however, life prolongation may not be desired if this is at a time when the illness is progressing rapidly, leading to greater dependency on carers and increasing difficulty communicating their wishes.

For patients who lack capacity

Medical decisions for patients who lack capacity are governed by the Mental Capacity Act.[10] The Act came into force in 2007. It provides a legal framework for decisions about treatment for patients who lack capacity. It bolsters what was always good practice but also introduces new laws relating to patient advocacy.

The five key statutory principles that underpin the legal requirements of the MCA[13] are outlined in Box 8.3.

BOX 8.3 The five key statutory principles of the MCA

1 A person must be assumed to have capacity unless it is established that they lack capacity.
2 A person is not to be treated as unable to make a decision unless all practicable steps to help him to do so have been taken without success.

3 A person is not to be treated as unable to make a decision merely because he makes an unwise decision.

4 An act done, or decision made, under this Act for or on behalf of a person who lacks capacity must be done, or made, in his best interests.

5 Before the act is done, or the decision is made, regard must be had to whether the purpose for which it is needed can be as effectively achieved in a way that is less restrictive of the person's rights and freedom of action.

The Act details a two-stage test of capacity.[14] A lack of capacity is determined as follows.

1 There must be an impairment of the mind or brain.

2 There must be a failure to do at least one of the following:
   - comprehend the information given about a particular decision that needs to be made
   - retain that information for long enough to make a decision
   - weigh the information as part of the decision making process
   - communicate their decision by whatever means.

Capacity is decision-specific, i.e. a patient with an impairment of the mind may have capacity to make some decisions but not others depending on the level of complexity of the decisions involved and this may also vary over time.

All those involved in a person's care make assessments about that person's competence on a daily basis. Decisions such as what to have for breakfast, to have a wash, what clothes to wear etc. will be appropriately assessed by the carer assisting the person. However, where medical decisions, and particularly those of a serious nature, need to be made, more formal assessment should be made and documented. It is good practice for institutions caring for individuals with reduced capacity, such as hospitals and care homes to produce policies and procedures to support staff and protect the people in their care. Written documentation of the proposed decision and the person assessing capacity should be recorded.

Patients can make an Advance Decision to Refuse Treatment (ADRT) (*see* Box 8.4) while they still have capacity which would allow their wishes to be respected should they lose capacity at a later point. This would allow them to extend a degree of autonomy despite losing capacity.

BOX 8.4 Advance Decisions to Refuse Treatment (ADRTs)[15]

An ADRT enables someone aged 18 and over to refuse specified medical treatment for a time in the future when they may lack capacity to consent to or refuse treatment.

An ADRT only comes into force once the patient has lost capacity. The patient can cancel the ADRT at any time while they still have capacity.

An ADRT is legally binding if it meets the standards of validity and applicability laid out in the Mental Capacity Act 2005.

An ADRT is only binding for refusals of treatment, not requests for treatment.

A patient may produce an ADRT that is not valid and/or applicable and is therefore not legally binding. However, the health professional should still take into account what is set out in it when considering the patient's prior known wishes when making a best interests decision.

For patients with neurological conditions where lack of capacity is anticipated and a specific medical problem can also be reasonably anticipated, an ADRT gives the person the opportunity of influencing the decision making at that time. For instance, a patient with Huntington's disease will inevitably lose capacity as the disease progresses and is likely to become unable to manage food intake orally. The person may wish to make an advance decision before that time refusing tube feeding. If deemed valid and applicable at the time of presentation then it would be unlawful for a medical practitioner to initiate tube feeding. ADRTs may enable patients to extend their autonomy and also promote a greater sense of control over their future. However, it may be difficult for people to truly anticipate how they might feel in a particular circumstance in the future and this has to be borne in mind when discussing these with patients.

Some patients may choose to appoint someone with Lasting Power of Attorney for Personal Welfare who would be able to consent to or refuse medical treatment on the patient's behalf should they lose to capacity to make these decisions themselves (*see* Box 8.5).

BOX 8.5 Lasting Power of Attorney (LPA)[16]

A LPA is a legal document that allows a patient to give authority to someone else to make decisions about their welfare on their behalf. This includes the power to give or refuse consent to medical treatments, and even life prolonging treatments, if the patient has specified this.

A LPA will only come into force when the patient has lost capacity for the decision that needs to be made.

An attorney must always act in the best interests of the patient. An attorney cannot demand treatments that are not considered clinically appropriate.

For patients who lack capacity who do not have an LPA or legally binding ADRT then a 'best interests' decision will have to be taken. This should involve consultation with the multidisciplinary team and also those interested in the patient's welfare (i.e. family and friends). It can be a very difficult task to work out what is in someone's best interests and can be subject to bias if care is not taken. The MCA requires people to follow certain steps to help them work out what is in someone else's best interests. For more information see the Code of Practice.[17]

Medical treatments (including those that are potentially life prolonging) can be withheld or withdrawn if this is felt to be in the patient's best interests.

CASE EXAMPLE 8.2 Mr B

Mr B, aged 76, has advanced Parkinson's disease and is also profoundly demented. He is admitted to hospital having fallen out of bed at home and his wife is struggling to care for him on her own. He is bed bound and needs help with all care. His speech has become very limited and mainly consists of occasional moaning-like sounds. He is unable to communicate via any communication aid. While he is on the ward he stops taking any food or fluids by mouth. Any attempts to provide even small amounts of fluid either results in aspiration or Mr B becoming distressed. He is assessed by a speech and language therapist who confirms that he is unable to swallow even small amounts. The medical team attempts to put up a drip to provide fluids while they are deciding on a way forward but Mr B becomes very distressed each time during the procedure and the cannula becomes dislodged. He also often becomes agitated during his wash and cares. He has also not been able to tolerate a catheter at home and has pulled out several. The consultant is asked to review the patient to decide on the way forward. Should attempts be made to provide artificial nutrition and hydration (ANH) via a PEG (percutaneous endoscopic gastrostomy)? There appears to be some disagreement among the staff as to the correct way forward and also among his own family. One staff nurse on the ward round comments that 'It's wrong to let him starve to death.'

As mentioned in Box 8.2, ANH is considered medical treatment as a matter of law. It can, therefore, be withheld or withdrawn if it is not considered to be in the patient's best interests to provide it. An exception is when a person is in a persistent vegetative state when a legal ruling is needed.

What issues should the consultant consider in this situation?

- Does Mr B have capacity?
- Who should decide whether to provide ANH?
- What is in the patient's best interests?

Mr B is profoundly demented and does not have capacity to make decisions about ANH. He does not have an Advance Decision to Refuse Treatment,

Advance Statement of Preferences, Lasting Power of Attorney or a court appointed deputy. Under the Mental Capacity Act 2005 (MCA), therefore, the consultant ultimately has the responsibility of deciding whether attempts should be made to place a PEG feeding tube to provide ANH. He has to decide what is in the best interests of Mr B.

Respect for autonomy is difficult in this situation as Mr B lacks capacity. However, those close to the patient may be able to provide some insight into Mr B's former wishes and values. In terms of beneficence and non malefi-cence the consultant needs to consider what would be the benefits and harms of proceeding or not proceeding with PEG placement.

These sorts of complex and difficult decisions are best not taken alone. It is always vital to discuss the issues as a multidisciplinary team and to try to reach a consensus as to what is in the patient's best interests. It is also essential to get the insights and perspective of those close to the patient (and in fact this is a legal requirement under the MCA). Given that there has been some disagreement about how to proceed, the consultant organises a case conference with relevant staff and family members to discuss the relevant issues and to try to reach a consensus as to what is in the patient's best interests.

Would ANH prolong life in this situation and if so what would be the possible effects for Mr B? This is not easy to predict. Mr B is clearly at a very advanced stage of his illness and his prognosis is likely very short with or without ANH. However, it is quite likely that providing ANH will prolong Mr B's life. The burdens of ANH would appear to be considerable. He already becomes distressed by physical contact during cares and resists attempts at catheterisation and cannulation. His wife feels that he takes no obvious pleasure or meaning in his situation and that he has no apparent awareness of his family or of his surroundings. She feels that Mr B would not want ANH under the current circumstances. The consultant asks the local consultant neurologist who has previously been involved in Mr B's care for a second opinion.

After a full discussion of the above issues, it is decided by the consultant that it would not be in Mr B's best interests to provide ANH. The rest of the staff and family are in agreement. Mr B receives best symptomatic care to maintain his dignity and comfort. Mr B dies 10 days later peacefully with his family around him.

DEALING WITH DISPUTES UNDER THE MCA

There may be times when people disagree over aspects of decision making for patients who lack capacity. For instance, there may be a dispute about whether a patient actually has capacity or not, or over what is actually in the patient's best interests. It is obviously in everyone's interests to try to resolve disagreements as quickly and effectively as possible. The MCA Code of Practice outlines the process in detail.[18]

When health professionals are in dispute with a patient's relatives there are several strategies that may be helpful:

➤ make every effort to communicate as clearly and effectively as possible the different options and proposed way forward including the option of a case conference
➤ offer a second opinion
➤ involve an independent mediator.

In some cases, especially where the decision is of a particularly serious nature, an application to the Court of Protection may need to be made to resolve the issue.

CASE EXAMPLE 8.3 Mr C

Mr C is a 61 year old gentleman with motor neurone disease (MND). One of his carers found him unwell on Monday morning. He had been coughing over the weekend and had a temperature. She called for an ambulance and by the time he arrived in the A&E department he was drowsy and had difficulty breathing. His blood gases indicated respiratory failure, with pH 7.15, pO_2 8, pCO_2 11.2. He has a wife, who has taken a short holiday to visit their son in Spain. She has been contacted by the carer and is on her way home. He relies on a wheelchair, but was known to live independently at home with the support of his wife and carers. His carer was aware that he had been seen at a specialist hospital recently to be assessed for non invasive ventilation.

The intensive therapy consultant assesses Mr C for ventilation and ITU care.

- Does Mr C have capacity to decide about his ongoing treatment?
- Who should decide what is in his best interest?
- What is in his best interest?

Mr C, drowsy from a chest infection and resulting respiratory failure, probably does not have capacity, but this may well be reversible if his underlying condition is successfully treated. The decision to treat needs to be taken urgently as Mr C's condition is deteriorating. There is no known ADRT to consult, no Advance Statement of Preferences and no LPA. The obligation to consult anyone with an interest in Mr C's condition may be limited by the restricted time available. The ITU consultant must consider the chances of successfully treating Mr C and the likely ongoing sequelae after ITU care. In this circumstance treatment of his chest infection has a good chance of success but Mr C may well end up ventilator dependent, through a tracheostomy.

In the absence of any previously known wishes of Mr C, preservation of life is likely to be considered in his best interests. Successfully treating Mr C maximises his capacity, creating an opportunity for him to be involved in decision making in the future.

Mr C is taken to ITU, ventilated and treated with antibiotics. His wife returns from holiday and confirms that he had not made any advance decisions or statements and he had struggled with the idea of non invasive ventilation. His ITU stay is quite protracted due to developing further sepsis. Attempts to wean him off ventilation fail and his motor function declines. Three weeks later he is stable enough to be transferred to a ward. His communication is limited but with a letter board he indicates he does not want to continue with this existence. His tracheostomy tube frequently blocks and he finds suction very distressing. He asks for the ventilation to be switched off. Some members of the team looking after him find this request very difficult; his wife and others accept his decision. There is concern he may be depressed and therefore his capacity impaired. A psychiatric opinion is sought. In the meantime he develops a further overwhelming sepsis. After discussion between his wife and son and the multidisciplinary team it is decided that, this time, escalating treatment is not in his best interests as it is now unlikely to return him to a quality of life he would value. He dies three days later.

SUMMARY

We began this chapter by outlining how important ethical decision making is in healthcare. Medical decision making for patients with PLTNCs may present many ethical considerations as we have illustrated in this chapter. It is essential the multidisciplinary team works together with the patient and the family, not just to provide care and information but to listen to their worries and concerns. It is important to give the patient the opportunity to prepare for what might lie ahead. A good knowledge of the patient's condition including its prognosis and likely future course, as well as skilled communication and compassion are essential for health professionals if they are to help patients make decisions and if they are to be able to introduce the subject of advance care planning and, in so doing, preserve the patient's autonomy.

For patients who lack capacity, health professionals have to decide what is in their best interests. This can be a grave responsibility and can be subject to prejudice if particular care is not taken. The MCA requires a very specific process to be followed when assessing best interests which includes the duty to consult the patient's family and loved ones.

While it is difficult to do justice to such a complex topic in this chapter alone, we hope that we have provided a window into this challenging area and a basis for further reading about and exploration of the issues involved.

REFERENCES

1 Beauchamp T, Childress J. *Principles of Biomedical Ethics*. 5th ed. New York: Oxford University Press; 2001.
2 R (on the application of Burke) v General Medical Council (2004) EWCH 1879 (Admin).
3 General Medical Council. *Withdrawing and Withholding Life-prolonging Treatments: good practice in decision-making*. London: GMC; 2002.
4 British Medical Association. *Withholding and Withdrawing Life-prolonging Medical Treatment: guidance for decision making*. 3rd ed. London: BMJ Publishing Group; 2007.
5 R (on the application of Burke) v General Medical Council [2005] EWCA Civ 1003.
6 R (on the application of Burke) v General Medical Council, op. cit. at 34.
7 R (on the application of Burke) v General Medical Council, op. cit. at 31.
8 R (on the application of Burke) v General Medical Council, op. cit. at 32.
9 R (on the application of Burke) v General Medical Council, op. cit. at 50.
10 Mental Capacity Act 2005, (c9).
11 General Medical Council. *Consent: patients and doctors making decisions together*. London: GMC; 2008.
12 Leigh P, *et al*. The management of MND. *J Neurol Neurosurg Psychiatry*. 2003; 74(Suppl. IV): S32–47.
13 Department for Constitutional Affairs (DCA). *Mental Capacity Act 2005 Code of Practice* (2007 Final Edition). London: TSO. Chapter 2.
14 DCA. *Mental Capacity Act 2005 Code of Practice*, op. cit. Chapter 4.
15 DCA. *Mental Capacity Act 2005 Code of Practice*, op. cit. Chapter 9.
16 DCA. *Mental Capacity Act 2005 Code of Practice*, op. cit. Chapter 7.
17 DCA. *Mental Capacity Act 2005 Code of Practice*, op. cit. Chapter 5.
18 DCA. *Mental Capacity Act 2005 Code of Practice*, op. cit. Chapter 15.

Bereavement support

Aimee Aubeeluck and Elaine Duro

'He used to be loving and loveable but now that's all gone.'

Extract from Korer and Fitzsimmons (1985, p. 586)[1]

The experience of loss is a continuous process for all those affected by life limiting illness and, for people with progressive long-term neurological conditions (PLTNCs) and their family carers, one that can extend over many years prior to bereavement. This chapter will explore the experience of loss and bereavement and the intersection between the experiences of loss and bereavement and family care giving.

DEATH IN MODERN SOCIETY

The End of Life Care Strategy recently published by the Department of Health[2] suggests that dying and death are rarely discussed within modern society and that this lack of openness has resulted in people experiencing a significant level of fear and anxiety in relation to the processes of dying, death and bereavement. Yet even in modern developed societies individuals may be faced with the prospect of death across their lifespan. This is a phenomenon related to the very nature of our existence as humans[3] and can be viewed as both 'a reality and part of our culture',[4] even though most deaths occur in institutions such as hospitals and care homes and are removed from direct everyday experience of life for most of us.[5] When there is a lack of either public or professional discussion, individuals affected by long-term conditions which they know are likely to eventually contribute to or cause death (such as PLTNCs) are likely to feel particularly isolated.

When individuals are faced with the prospect of their own mortality or that of someone to whom they are close, once taken-for-granted assumptions about the world are challenged and life may, often unexpectedly, take on a new and very fragile form.[6] Yet if understanding and acceptance of the inevitability of loss and mortality could be adopted and demonstrated in practice and in daily life, enormous benefits could be established. Those facing death could more easily make their final wishes known and their families and friends would be able to express what this loss means for them and their future.[7] It has been argued that 'it is valuable to talk, but it is even more comforting to be heard by someone who appears to recognize that need to talk and appreciates it is hard to do so'.[8]

BEREAVEMENT AND LOSS

The word 'bereavement' is derived from the verb 'bereave', which means to 'rob, dispossess of, leave desolate, and deprive of a relationship',[9] and is a term frequently used to describe loss from death of someone significant within a person's life.[10] Bereavement is viewed as challenging a person's sense of identity, but is generally 'socially managed' by the bereaved in ways that cause least disturbance to society.[11] The word 'grief' primarily describes a person's emotional response to loss, particularly where the loss relates to that of an emotionally important figure.[12] Among those who grieve the loss of someone who has died, a 'sense of limbo' may be experienced, which can persist for some years until the individual makes sense of, and adjusts to, their new status as a bereaved person. Grief can be viewed as the emotional cost associated with recognising the finality of the loss of a loved one.[13] The term 'mourning' denotes the social context and behaviour surrounding the expression of grief (for example, the ways in which funeral ceremonies are carried out) and may be shaped and influenced by predominant cultural mores.[14]

It has been argued that bereavement has for individuals some of the most powerful and far reaching consequences of any life event. It may be likened to entering a 'foreign country',[15] whereby the overwhelming experience is of disorientation: familiar relationships are transformed and the individual feels a sense of helplessness.[16] Bereavement has been associated with a decline in survivors' physical and mental health.[17] As such, there is an emphasis on the use of research findings to inform practice,[18] with the aim of improving bereavement care and enhancing quality of life for bereaved survivors.[19]

Much of the experience of illness is associated with a continuous experience of loss for what may be many years prior to death and bereavement: loss of independence, ability to work, social roles that may be highly valued, or the loss of many other less obvious aspects of daily life. Among those affected by neurological conditions, losses such as the ability to walk unaided or to express oneself verbally, or loss of the ability to express emotions or to control emotions, may be particularly hard to bear. Such losses are experienced not only by the person with the PLTNC, but also by those close to them: particularly their families. Loss of income, of future plans and changes in relationships are all features of a life lived with loss for those affected by PLTNCs. For those who care for a person with a progressive neurological condition, loss becomes bound up with the experience of care giving and where care giving is done without adequate help and support it can have profound effects on the subsequent experience of bereavement.

THEORIES RELATED TO BEREAVEMENT AND GRIEF

Our understanding of loss and bereavement, especially in relation to death and dying, has been greatly influenced by the concepts of attachment and separation. The characterisation of bonds or broken bonds has informed many models of bereavement, theories and grief resolution.[20] Moreover, recent research has argued that the 'presence' of the dead, plays an important moral role in the lives of the living.[21] Such generalised theories seek to provide an explanatory framework that describes a broad range of phenomena and consequences created by the experience of bereavement. Table 9.1 provides a generalised summary of how theorists have perceived the phenomenon of grief and individuals' reactions to this life changing event. This table has incorporated a broad range of theoretical bereavement models, designed to explain the process of grief. It is important to be aware that while these are helpful in enabling thought about the issues of relevance, there is no single 'correct' or 'true' theory that explains the experience of loss and bereavement.

TABLE 9.1 Theory of grief and individuals' reactions

Parkes' Theory of Grief (Parkes 1972)[22]	Considers that grief is a 'pre-programmed' sequence of behaviours within individuals. During the early stage of the grief process, the inner representations of the deceased are an important element to the living. This model goes on to propose that once grief resolution has been achieved, interaction with the 'dead' serves no useful purpose.
The Two Track Model (Rubin 1981)[23]	Examines the phenomenon of death by assuming that it comprises of two tracks. Track I relates to the bereaved person's bio-psychosocial reaction towards the bereavement. Track II focuses upon the attachment relationship with the deceased. This model illustrates how death transforms a relationship and leads the living to adopt a new ongoing relationship to the deceased.
The Task Model (Worden 1982)[24]	Presents grieving in terms of 'tasks' that a bereaved person must perform in order to adjust to bereavement. Thus the griever actively works through the grief process, rather than just passively experiencing it.

(continued)

Walter's New Model of Grief (Walter 1996)[25]	Proposes that the function of grief permits the bereaved to grasp the reality of death. This is achieved by constructing a 'durable biography' of the deceased, which the living can integrate into their lives.
The Model of Incremental Grief (Cook & Oltjenbruns 1998)[26]	Indicates than one loss can trigger another. This results in intensifying the grief process with each added loss. Suggests that bereavement may lead to 'secondary loss' within an individual's life. Thus a change can occur between grievers within a relationship.
The Dual Process Model (Stroebe & Schut 1999)[27]	This model seeks to integrate existing bereavement ideas and suggests that bereavement is a dynamic coping process in which oscillation may transpire within bereaved individuals. At times individuals will confront loss, while at other times it may be avoided.

GRIEF

The terms bereavement and grief are often used interchangeably, with bereavement being a term used to describe the 'objective reality of loss' and grief being the individual's feelings (which may be hidden) about this loss.[28] The individual's experiences of bereavement and grief are linked to the nature of their relationship or attachment to the deceased person. Grief has been described as the emotions associated with the individual's adjustment to undesirable world changes[29] and may involve anxiety, anger, yearning and pining.[30] A complex interplay of interpersonal, cultural and psychodynamic factors[31] contributes to the individual's experience of grief and manifests with physical, affective, cognitive, spiritual reactions.[32] The grieving process has been compared to a roller coaster in which bereaved individuals become enveloped in a cycle of fluctuating emotions.[33] Some people experience overwhelming emotions which can reappear on anniversaries such as birthdays or other special dates attributed to the deceased, sometimes for many years after the initial loss.

Martin and Doka (2000)[34] suggest that there may be two distinct patterns of grief – intuitive and instrumental – with a third pattern of dissonance being a combination of both (*see* Box 9.1). Intuitive grief is the manifestation of the expression of spontaneous, profoundly painful feelings that need to be shared. During the process of instrumental grief such feelings become tempered; and grief ultimately becomes more of an 'intellectual' experience. Martin and Doka[35] suggest that patterns of grief usually exist along a continuum and are influenced by gender, culture, and an individual's temperament. They argue that in Western culture men are likely to be found on the instrumental end of this continuum whereas women are likely to be found on the intuitive end: this may be due to powerful cultural mores shaping behaviour and subjective experience. However, they also note that many individuals may show blended patterns of behaviour and use a range of emotional, behavioural, and cognitive strategies to adapt to loss.

BOX 9.1 Martin and Doka's (2000)[34] two distinct patterns of grief

The intuitive griever	The instrumental griever
Feelings are experienced intensely	Thinking is foremost and feelings are less intense
	There is a general reluctance to talk about feelings
Expressed emotions, e.g. crying	Control over oneself and the environment
Adaptive strategies aid the experience and expression of feelings	Problem solving aids mastery of feelings and environment
Prolonged periods of confusion, inability to concentrate, disorganization and disorientation	Brief periods of cognitive dysfunction, confusion, forgetfulness, obsessive behaviour
Physical exhaustion and anxiety	Enhanced energy levels, no obvious symptoms of general grief reactions

CONTINUING BONDS IN BEREAVEMENT

The classical viewpoint on maintaining a bond with the deceased suggests that successful mourning requires the bereaved to emotionally 'detach' themselves from the person who has died.[36] However, at the beginning of the 21st century, we recognise the complexity of human nature and the importance of interdependence in our lives.[37] Psychological theories of grief have always had their roots firmly located within the attachment relationship between the survivor and the deceased.[38] Hence if individuals are able to mentally evoke a representation of this attachment figure, they experience a feeling of security.[39] Thus significant relationships can be represented in the mind's eye[40] and as such the internalised presence of the deceased allows the bereaved to become emotionally sustained.[41] Research has concluded that even those who are well adjusted to bereavement may experience an ongoing sense of presence of the deceased (in dreams for example), which provides them with some comfort.[42]

Some experts, such as Shaver and Tancredy (2001),[43] acknowledge the role of continuing bonds within the bereavement process[44] and recognise that it is part of normal experience to 'hold' memories of the deceased person for long periods of time[45] such that the inner representation of the deceased person becomes a living legacy and an active part of the life of those left behind.[46] This continuing bond between the living and the dead may allow some bereaved people to consider that the dead person resides in 'another plane'.[47] Dreams, memories and conversations about the deceased are all elements that permit the mourner to continue a connection to this dead person.

CARE GIVING, LOSS AND BEREAVEMENT

As views of bereavement evolve, there is a growing recognition of the complexity of human nature and the complexity and importance of relationships in people's lives. Current thinking in bereavement support acknowledges the need for the bereaved to have a continuing bond with the dead person and advocates that the quality of the relationship prior to death enables this ongoing connection after death.[48] However, successful navigation through the bereavement process may be difficult for family members of people with PLTNCs. The impact of the disease may be overwhelming for individuals and their families and their relationships may suffer. For example, within families affected by the genetically inherited disorder Huntington's disease (HD) younger family members are often aware that they may develop the illness for years before there are any noticeable symptoms; this may lead to anger and resentment. In other conditions, coping with profound personality changes may be experienced as challenging and extremely difficult. Such issues may only be the tip of the iceberg in terms of carers' needs and the associated complexities of loss. The emotional impact of care provision on the family carer, the need for support and the development of coping mechanisms in order to deal with inevitable bereavement are all important areas to consider when reflecting upon bereavement issues in neurological disorders.

AN EXAMPLE OF ISSUES IN FAMILY CARE PROVISION IN HUNTINGTON'S DISEASE (HD)

Family members play a leading role in homecare for the individual with a neurological disorder.[49] Indeed, Cantor (1983)[50] and Johnson (1983)[51] argue that help from the 'informal network' (i.e. partners, children, other relatives, friends and neighbours) is the most important source of support. Moreover, caring for a family member with a progressive illness appears to be unique in the challenges it creates for the family caregiver. Hans and Gilmore (1968)[52] note the major emotional, social and financial problems that care giving in HD can create for the family. In a more recent study, Semple (1995)[53] also notes the psychosocial effects of HD on the family. In a qualitative study that explored and described the experiences of family members of individuals with HD, Semple found that family carers experience a wide range of negative emotions as a result of their care giving role and that this has a significant impact on their own well-being. It has been argued that such issues are made worse due to the lack of attention that HD has received from public health services in terms of interventions.

Patients and their families find enormous difficulty in gaining access to specific services. Service provision for HD families is therefore often poor and unsuitable so families are mostly burdened with the main responsibility of care.[54]

Tyler, *et al.* (1983)[55] examined the relationship between HD disease state, family breakdown and stress in a sample of 92 patients. They found that violence, promiscuity and bizarre behaviour (i.e. the behavioural manifestations of HD) were often reported to be the cause of marital breakdown in HD. Behavioural problems were also cited as one of the main causes of stress within the family, with dangerous and aggressive behaviour reported in nearly half of all patients and 82% of primary carers reporting feeling stressed. Wives also reported feelings of conflict in choosing between caring for their HD affected spouse and their children over the duration of the illness. Furthermore, Hans and Koeppen (1980)[56] argue that HD permeates the entire life of the non HD spouse (e.g. lifestyle, family responsibility, goals and marital relationships) and so they experience continuous loss and trauma. They found that once a diagnosis had been made, the spouse was often called upon to help in the management of the patient in terms of supervision, moral support, nursing (i.e. long-term and palliative care), handling of finances and total responsibility for the home and any children.

The mood and behavioural changes associated with HD can drastically alter family, and especially spousal, relationships. Hans and Koeppen's (1980)[57] qualitative study of 15 wives of individuals with HD found that partners frequently describe the way in which they feel they have ended up married to a different person and perhaps not the sort of person they would have chosen. Feelings of regret, anger and ambivalence are commonplace and often marriages come under extreme pressure. Furthermore, as the partners became aware of the steady progression of the disease process and the threat of disease transmission to any children, they became resentful and hostile. The strain on members of the family is therefore further intensified by the impact of the unique implications stemming from the inherited nature of the disease.[58]

Because of the genetic implications of HD, it impacts upon individual family members in different ways. Spousal carers who have children have to deal with the possibility that their children may also be carrying the HD gene. This puts them in a position where they could be caring for affected loved ones over a number of generations on top of having to cope with the possibility of resentment towards their spouse for putting them in this situation. Children and other family members who are carers may have to cope with either an 'at risk' HD gene-positive or HD gene-negative status thus giving them the possibility of watching how they themselves may deteriorate in the future or what they have been saved from. These different carer roles are therefore very distinct with regards to the burden that they may place onto individual carers as they provide palliative care for their loved ones.

DEALING WITH STRESS AND LEARNING TO COPE WITH LOSS

Most current care giving research is built on stress and coping or stress-process models in order to understand the impact of care giving. Lazarus and Folkman (1984)[59] argue that an individual may engage in a number of coping strategies in order to reduce the adverse emotional state associated with the appraisal of (perceived) stress. These fall into the two categories of problem focused and emotion focused coping (*see* Box 9.2). The goal of both strategies is for the individual to control their level of stress. In problem focused coping people try to short-circuit negative emotions by taking some action to modify, avoid, or minimise the threatening situation, i.e. the individual attempts to change the situation in order to reduce its threat. In emotion focused coping people try to directly moderate or eliminate unpleasant emotions without actually trying to change the situation. Examples of emotion focused coping include rethinking the situation in a positive way, relaxation, denial, and wishful thinking. A number of more specific categories are subsumed within these two broad categories as outlined here.

Both types of coping can occur simultaneously[60] and the success of any effort depends on the individual involved and the nature of the challenge. In general, problem focused coping is the most effective coping strategy when people have realistic opportunities to change aspects of their situation and reduce stress. Emotion focused coping is most useful as a short-term strategy. It can help reduce one's arousal level before engaging in problem solving and taking action, and it can help people deal with stressful situations in which there are few problem focused coping options. The model focuses on coping processes that can be used to manage or reduce aversive states. However, it is also based on the assumption that an event is not stressful unless the individual perceives it to be stressful.[61]

BOX 9.2 Examples of problem focused and emotion focused coping from Lazarus and Folkman's (1984) stress-coping model

Problem focused coping	**Emotion focused coping**
Confrontive coping	Distancing
Seeking social support	Self control
Planful problem solving	Positive reappraisal
Accepting responsibility	Escape/avoidance

This model, when applied to care giving in neurological disorders, places emphasis on the carer to re-interpret their situation as non threatening. For carers who are already overburdened, this added pressure may be overwhelming. Furthermore, within a chronic and palliative care giving situation there may be very little realistic opportunity to change any aspect of their situation. Indeed, for family carers of patients with long-term conditions, it is probable that the stressors they encounter are likely to increase throughout the duration of their care giving role as the burden 'mounts up' over the course of time.[62]

A model that may be more pertinent to family carers providing long-term palliative care comes from Pearlin, et al. (1990)[63] who developed a framework that allows the demands and resources of the caregiver to be clearly identified. They distinguish four domains: background and contextual factors; stressors; mediators of stress; and outcomes. The stressors are themselves divided into three types: primary stressors, directly connected with providing care; secondary role strains such as those caused by the conflicting demands of caring, work and family; and secondary intra-psychic strains, including the impact of caring on self esteem. They have further developed an interview schedule to pick up the major factors within each of these domains. This particular framework accounts for many influential factors such as culture and life history. Other mediating factors include resources for coping with social, economic and internal stresses. The schedule provides a clear system for outlining a carer's situation and can also be used to suggest relevant interventions. The model is outlined in Figure 9.1.

The purpose of considering palliative family care giving in relation to stress and coping is to gain understanding that may help to prevent or ameliorate stress related problems and enable the carer to continue providing palliative care comfortably for their relative (assuming that this is what both would wish) while dealing with their loss over time and coping with death when it comes. Stress process models demonstrate possible areas for intervention at the level of reducing primary or secondary stressors, working to address intra-psychic

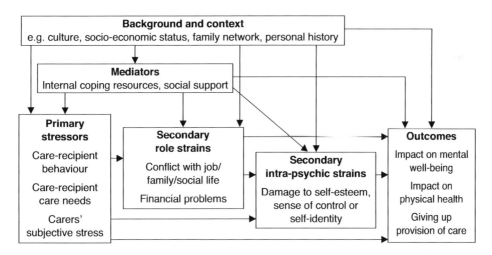

FIGURE 9.1 Pearlin's stress process model of stress in carers. Adapted from: Pearlin, et al.; 1990.[63]

strain or improving mediators such as coping skills or social support. The main treatment strategies include: the provision of information; assistance with problem solving to manage stressors; and providing or identifying sources of emotional and practical support. The modalities include one-to-one counselling or therapy; family meetings; and support groups. Although these may sound straightforward and almost common sense, in practice they may be complex because of the intertwined emotional and practical issues involved. For example, a person who attributes a HD relative's behaviourally rigid behaviour (i.e. getting stuck in an idea or task) to their personality may require information about the nature of the brain and executive function. However, they may be emotionally defended against the knowledge that their relative is getting progressively worse so getting the information across in a sensitive yet useful way can take time and be difficult to achieve.

BOX 9.3 An outline of caregiver concerns in relation to palliative family care giving in neurological disorders

	Bereavement/Loss
Chronic nature of neurological disorders	Loss of caregiver's life to an extended palliative care giving role
Symptomology	Person is no longer as they once were and grief may come before death
	Death may come as a relief
	Relationship may be damaged which could impact on 'continuing bond'
Genetic implications (especially in Huntington's disease)	Spousal carers who have children may care for affected loved ones over a number of generations leading to loss/grief over children's health status
	Children and other family members who are carers may have to cope with either an 'at risk' or HD gene-positive status giving them the possibility of watching how they themselves may deteriorate and leading to grief for their own life

The need to support family caregivers of people with PLTNCs in providing care is clear. The progressive nature of such disorders means that the caregiver role is always evolving and creating new problems/challenges, always associated with loss for carers; often over a long period of time. How carers cope and adjust to their ever changing role may depend on how stressors are perceived and interpreted.[64] However, it is important to note that for carers in a chronic care giving situation there may be very little realistic opportunity to change any aspect of their situation.

Moreover, there are a number of issues with neurological conditions that may complicate the bereavement process and may make coping with loss particularly distressing (*see* Box 9.3). The duration of the illness and the multitude of symptoms may mean that bereavement comes long before death itself. This may be especially difficult within a spousal relationship in the sense that an intimate and loving bond may no longer exist but, unlike a bereavement caused by death, the person is living with them as a constant reminder of that lost relationship.[65]

WHO IS AT RISK IN BEREAVEMENT?

'Bereavement is a darkness impenetrable to the imagination of the unbereaved.'

Iris Murdoch[66]

Sheldon (1998)[67] has identified a number of factors that increase the risk of a poor outcome in bereavement. One particular factor that may leave family caregivers of neurological patients at greater risk is the impact that the disease process may have had on the patient–caregiver relationship. It is argued that the living relationship with the deceased person is a significant factor in gaining an adaptive outcome in the bereavement process. Ambivalent or dependent relationships are linked with higher distress, regardless of whether it was the person who died or the person bereaved who was overtly dependent on the other. With a neurological disorder it is likely that the person who died will have become highly dependent on the bereaved as they will have been providing palliative nursing care to their loved one. Furthermore, the strain of caring for a terminally ill person for longer than six months is associated with an increased risk of poor outcome after death. It has been suggested by Relf, *et al.* (2008)[68] that family members frequently focus their energy upon the dying person during the latter stage of the palliative care process; in many cases relatives are unwilling to explore and evaluate their own needs related to this challenging life changing event during this time. Hence an individual's resilience and vulnerability within 'bereavement resolve' may be influenced and shaped by circumstantial factors as indicated earlier within this chapter, namely: relationship difficulties, the difficulty of the loved one's death, financial hardship and housing problems. Thus it should be considered that the manifestation of feeling overwhelmed within the grief process is viewed as being greater and more persistent if the individual is privy to these types of stressful life demands. Accordingly, one's own personal resourcefulness can become somewhat limited when such circumstantial demands become so high within life. This leads individuals to become prone to distress and tension as they struggle to maintain control of their lives while attempting to hold their distressing powerful emotions of grief at bay. Accordingly, bereaved individuals become less self confident and optimistic when dealing with the effects of this life changing event.

A person's normal strategies for remaining in control of their lives can become easily defeated during bereavement situations, leading such people to become overwhelmed by feelings of anxiety following the death of their loved one. Furthermore, bereaved individuals who perceive their social support as lacking are also more at risk; therefore it is important that bereavement services are made readily available during the very early stages of bereavement resolve to individuals who are deemed to have 'high' levels of vulnerability within their daily lives. Box 9.4 summarises these points.

BOX 9.4 Risk factors for poor outcomes in bereavement and implications for long-term family carers

Risk factors associated with poor outcomes in bereavement	Implications for long-term family carers
Ambivalent or dependent relationship	Relationship likely to be both ambivalent and dependent due to the nature of symptomology and disease progression
Multiple prior bereavements	Always a possibility (especially in HD due to its genetic nature)
Previous mental illness, especially depression	Research links depression to long-term care giving
Low self esteem of bereaved person	Isolation/loss of spousal relationship/care giving role may lead to low self esteem
Untimely death of young person	Possible (especially in cases of juvenile HD)
Stigmatised deaths – such as AIDS, suicide	Some individuals still experience stigma in relation to neurological conditions
Culpable deaths	No real culpability although families may experience a feeling of responsibility
Caring for deceased person for over 6 months	Likely to have been care giving for a number of years.
Level of perceived social support	Many caregivers report feelings of isolation and lack of social support
Lack of opportunities for new interests	These may be limited as carer may be required to care for other family members

SUPPORTING THE BEREAVED

In palliative care, only a small number of deaths may be seen as sudden or unexpected by health professionals. However, it is important to remember that bereaved family and friends may hold a different view and even when death is expected that it can come as a shock. A number of measures can be taken to try and reduce the impact of death and encourage a positive outcome for family carers, which are summarised in Box 9.5.

BOX 9.5 Measures to reduce the impact of death

Some actions/interventions that may help family carers through the grieving process.
- Being present at the death, seeing the body afterwards, and attending the funeral or memorial service.
- Providing information about the feelings they may experience and sources of voluntary support through leaflets/empathetic personal contact.
- Bereavement counselling targeted at those in high risk categories.
- Bereavement support groups.

Families and carers have particular needs when they are faced with the demise of a loved one. Firstly, it is important to consider that people faced with a traumatic or threatening situation such as a PLTNC or impending bereavement may be affected by symptoms of psychological distress. These may range from sadness or worry, to distress which is so intense that it interferes with a person's ability to function on a day to day basis. For most people, grief is dealt with by individuals drawing upon their own inner resources and obtaining emotional support from family members or friends. However, some people find it too difficult or traumatic to respond and adapt to such a life changing transition without additional professional help. The appropriate level of psychological intervention a person might require is largely dependent upon the nature and severity of any psychological issue. The process of assessment for psychological intervention will consider whether the individual has experienced any previous psychological or mental health difficulties while establishing the quality of social support networks available to the person. Healthcare professionals offering day to day care are able to provide general psychological support to individuals and have a key role in assessing a person's psychological well-being. Accordingly, these professionals should be able to signpost individuals to more specialised services such as counselling, clinical and health psychology, liaison psychiatry and social work.

Box 9.6 outlines the specific needs and services that might be required to support bereaved people. We have drawn upon the most salient recommendations from the NICE (2004)[69] guidelines and added to these. We would suggest that such services are applicable to the bereavement needs of all individuals who are faced with the prospect of the demise of a loved one through long-term illness.

BOX 9.6 Amalgamation of NICE 2004 guidelines and our own recommendations for bereavement support

Professionals involved in the practice and delivery of supportive palliative and bereavement care should have access to regular and ongoing training to ensure their professional development is maintained within this culturally sensitive domain. Such practice should be considered as a mandatory requirement within this sphere of work, and therefore ought to be extended to doctors within general practice.

Health and social care professionals providing day to day support to family members and carers ought to initially assess and address the needs of these individuals, considering the family's coping ability, stress levels and available support. Such assessments should happen shortly after bereavement has occurred. Ongoing, proactive engagement should be endorsed by healthcare professionals for people who are considered to be at risk of psychological 'damage' following a significant or difficult bereavement.

Our multicultural society requires that the cultural and ethnic background of bereaved individuals is acknowledged during any psychological assessment process, and also considered within the remit of any form of intervention.

Bereavement services are required to be in place to meet the whole spectrum of needs of bereaved people. Differing types of support and relevant interventions ought to be offered within a reasonable timeframe to bereaved people. These services should also respect the long-term ongoing nature of bereavement resolve. Hence such services ought to be sufficiently resourced to fully provide this aspect of care.

Both family members and carers should be made aware of the information, advice and support networks available to them. They should be 'signposted' to both local and national sources of help and information, which are specifically designed to meet their own needs.

Bereaved individuals should be actively encouraged to seek and use existing support networks. If access to such support is insufficient to meet the needs of the individual, or if it is considered the grief reaction maybe be difficult for the person to experience, then access to additional help and support services should be made readily available to people.

CONCLUDING THOUGHTS

Modern society has undergone a rapid social change in which traditional family and community support networks are in fast decline; in some cases this means that there is a greater need of professional help and support at and around the time of death, which for some families will be experienced as a crisis.[70] Dying, death and bereavement pose a significant challenge to families and carers of the terminally ill[71] which, for some people, becomes a long lasting, haunting and inescapable dimension to their daily lives.[72] The demise of a loved one and the subsequent bereavement process may give rise to a variety of needs and challenges for the members of a family: practical, financial, emotional, social and spiritual.[73] Bereaved individuals have to gradually re-learn and re-prioritise their 'assumptions about the world . . . and [this] involves incorporating and re-interpreting the past rather than giv[ing] it up'.[74] While most bereaved people manage to find and access the resources that help them through this difficult time, others will require outside help with this process. There is no single intervention that will meet the needs of all bereaved people, but there is a range of resources which have been found to be helpful, including individual interviews, group sessions and telephone contact. Such services can be found within both the statutory and voluntary sectors. However, it has been suggested by Relf (2008)[75] that while bereavement support may be offered in many guises to bereaved individuals, the economic and human resources for such services are usually in 'short supply'. Such services are therefore obligated to make the best use of very limited resources within this domain. While it may be argued that many people within society may have the inner resources and social support of family and friends to be able to actively manage their bereavement distress following the death of a loved one, a substantial minority of bereaved individuals find it difficult to adjust to such a death and this can lead them to experience persisted physical and mental health problems. It should therefore be acknowledged that a person's need for supportive services during the bereavement process varies. Accordingly, the NICE 2004 guidelines[76] have advocated both the importance of offering information to bereaved individuals about this most complex and life changing of experiences and the importance of showing the bereaved how to gain access to the differing forms of support during the bereavement process. Accordingly, individual bereavement counselling has been shown to be particularly useful to individuals at risk of a poor outcome in bereavement[77] and may be useful in supporting bereaved family carers. Ultimately, listening attentively and actively to a distressed individual aids the person in articulating new meaning and promotes recovery.[78] When giving support to the bereaved it is important to take a flexible approach which incorporates the wishes of the individual as they rebuild their life. However, this process should not exclude the possibility of bereaved individuals enduring some level of continued distress over their entire lifespan, albeit at a much lower level than was initially experienced. While there is a notion that bereavement does resolve, a precise endpoint in time cannot be specified for bereaved individuals.[79] Klass (1997)[80] states that 'the grief is the price we pay for love' (p. 160). In successful bereavement resolution individuals undertake a major revision of their lives with long lasting, rather than transient, implications.[81]

'As a family we can get through whatever life's challenges are.'

Extract taken from Aubeeluck (2005)[82]

REFERENCES

1 Korer J, Fitzsimmons JS. The effect of Huntington's chorea on family life. *Br J Soc Work.* 1985; **15**: 581–97.
2 Department of Health. *End of Life Care Strategy: promoting high quality care for all adults at the end of life.* London: DH; 2008.
3 Leahy JM. A comparison of depression in women bereaved of a spouse, child or a parent. *Omega.* 1992; **26**(30): 207–17.
4 Wass H. A perspective on the current state of death education. *Death Stud.* 2004; **28**(4): 289–308.
5 Department of Health, op. cit.
6 Riches G, Dawson P. *An Intimate Loneliness: supporting bereaved parents and siblings.* Buckingham: Open University Press; 2000.
7 National Institute for Health and Clinical Excellence. *Guidance on Cancer Services: improving supportive and palliative care for adults with cancer: the manual.* London: NICE; 2004.
8 Riches G, op. cit.
9 Coulson J, Carr CT, Hutchinson L, *et al. The Oxford Illustrated Dictionary.* London: Book Club Associates; 1981.
10 Stroebe MS, Hansson RO, Stroebe W, *et al.* Introduction: concepts and issues in contemporary research on bereavement. In: Stroebe MS, Hansson RO, Stroebe W, *et al.*, editors. *Handbook of Bereavement Research: consequences, coping and care.* Washington, DC: American Psychological Association; 2001. pp. 3–22.
11 Riches G, op. cit.
12 Weiss RS. Grief, bonds and relationships. In: Stroebe MS, Hansson RO, Stroebe W, *et al.*, editors. *Handbook of Bereavement Research: consequences, coping and care.* Washington, DC: American Psychological Association; 2001. pp. 47–62.
13 Riches G, op. cit.
14 Stroebe MS, op. cit.
15 Zisook S. *Biopsychosocial Aspects of Bereavement.* Washington, DC: American Psychiatric Press; 1987.
16 Ibid.
17 Genevro JL, Marshall T, Miller T. Report on bereavement and grief research. *Death Stud.* 2004; **28**(6): 491–575.
18 Murphy SA. The use of research findings in bereavement programs: a case study. *Death Stud.* 2000; **24**(7): 585–602.

19 Raphael B, Minkov C, Dobson M. Psychotherapeutic and pharmacological intervention for bereaved persons. In: Stroebe MS, Hansson RO, Stroebe W, *et al.*, editors. *Handbook of Bereavement Research: consequences, coping and care.* Washington, DC: American Psychological Association; 2001. pp. 587–612.

20 Bruce EJ, Schultz C. *Non-finite Loss & Grief: a psycho-educational approach.* London: Jessica Kingsley Publishers; 2001.

21 Stroebe MS, *et al.*, op. cit.

22 Parkes CM. *Bereavement: studies of grief in adult life.* New York: International Universities Press; 1972.

23 Rubin S. A two-track model of bereavement: theory and application in research. *Am J Orthopsychiatry.* 1981; **51**: 101–9.

24 Worden W. *Grief Counselling and Grief Therapy: a handbook for the mental health practitioner.* New York: Springer; 1982.

25 Walter T. A new model of grief: bereavement and biography. *Mortality.* 1996; **1**: 7–25.

26 Cook A, Oltjenbruns K. *Dying and Grieving: lifespan and family perspectives.* Fort Worth, TX: Harcourt Brace; 1998.

27 Stroebe M, Schut H. The dual process model of coping with bereavement: rationale and description. *Death Stud.* 1999; **23**: 197–224.

28 Martin TL, Doka KJ. *Men Don't Cry . . . Women Do: transcending gender stereotypes of grief.* London: Brunner/Mazel; 2000.

29 Ibid.

30 Shaver PR, Tancredy CM. Emotion, attachment and bereavement: a conceptual commentary. In: Stroebe MS, Hansson RO, Stroebe W, *et al.*, editors. *Handbook of Bereavement Research: consequences, coping and care.* Washington, DC: American Psychological Association; 2001. pp. 63–88.

31 Thompson N. Introduction. In: Thompson N, editor. *Loss and Grief: a guide for human services practitioners.* Basingstoke: Palgrave; 2002. pp. 1–20.

32 Martin TL, op. cit.

33 Ibid.

34 Ibid.

35 Ibid.

36 Freud S. *Lines of Advance in Psycho-Analytic Therapy, Standard Edition, Vol. 17.* London: Hogarth Press; 1955.

37 Klass D. The deceased child in the psychic and social worlds of bereaved parents during the resolution of grief. *Death Stud.* 1997; **21**(2): 147–76.

38 Martin TL, op. cit.

39 Field NP, Goa B, Paderna L. Continuing bonds in bereavement: an attachment theory based perspective. *Death Stud.* 2005; **29**(4): 277–99.

40 Rubin SS, Malkin R. Parental response to child loss across the life cycle: clinical and research perspectives. In: Stroebe MS, Hansson RO, Stroebe W, *et al.*, editors. *Handbook of Bereavement Research: consequences, coping and care.* Washington, DC: American Psychological Association; 2001. pp. 219–40.

41 Field NP, *et al.*, op. cit.

42 Parkes CM, Weiss R. *Recovery from Bereavement.* New York: Basic Books Inc.; 1983.

43 Shaver PR, op. cit.

44 Klass D, Walter T. Processes of grieving: how bonds are continued. In: Stroebe MS,

Hansson RO, Stroebe W, *et al.*, editors. *Handbook of Bereavement Research: consequences, coping and care.* Washington, DC: American Psychological Association; 2001. pp. 431–48.

45 Silverman PR, Nickman SL. Concluding thoughts. In: Klass D, Silverman PR, Nickman SL, editors. *Continuing Bonds: new understandings of grief.* London: Taylor & Francis; 1996. pp. 349–55.

46 Normand CL, Silverman PR, Nickman SL. Bereaved children's changing relationships with the deceased. In: Klass D, Silverman PR, Nickman SL, editors. *Continuing Bonds: new understandings of grief.* London: Taylor & Francis; 1996. pp. 87–111.

47 Silverman PR, op. cit.

48 Ibid.

49 Kessler S. Forgotten person in the Huntington disease family. *Am J Med Genet.* 1993; **48**: 145–50.

50 Cantor M. Strain among caregivers: a study of experience in the United States. *Gerontologist.* 1983; **23**: 597–604.

51 Johnson C. Dyadic family relations and social support. *Gerontologist.* 1983; **27**: 377–83.

52 Hans MB, Gilmore TH. Social aspects of Huntington's chorea. *Br J Psychiatry.* 1968; **114**: 93–8.

53 Semple OD. The experiences of family members of persons with Huntington's disease. *Perspectives.* 1995; **19**(4): 4–10.

54 Shakespeare J, Anderson J. Huntington's disease – falling through the net. *Health Trends (England).* 1993; **25**(1): 19–23.

55 Tyler A, Harper PS, Davies K, *et al.* Family break-down and stress in Huntington's chorea. *J Biosoc Sci.* 1983; **15**: 127–38.

56 Hans MB, Koeppen AH. Huntington's chorea: its impact on the spouse. *J Nerv Ment Disord.* 1980; **168**: 209–14.

57 Ibid.

58 Williams JK, Schutte DL, Holkup PA, *et al.* Psychosocial impact of predictive testing for Huntington's disease on support persons. *Am J Med Genet (Neuropsychiatric Genetics).* 2000; **96**: 353–9.

59 Lazarus RS, Folkman S. *Stress, Appraisal and Coping.* New York: Springer; 1984.

60 Folkman S, Lazarus RS. An analysis of coping in a middle-aged community sample. *J Health Soc Behav.* 1980; **21**: 219–39.

61 Tomaka J, Blascovich J, Kibler J, *et al.* Cognitive and physiological antecedents of threat and challenge appraisal. *J Pers Soc Psychol.* 1997; **73**: 63–72.

62 George LK, Gwyther LP. *The dynamics of caregiver-burden: changes in caregiver well-being over time.* Paper presented at the Annual Meeting of the Gerontological Society of America, San Antonio; 1984.

63 Pearlin LI, Mullan JT, Semple SJ, *et al.* Caregiving and the stress process: an overview of the concepts and their measures. *Gerontologist.* 1990; **30**: 583–93.

64 Lazarus RS, op. cit.

65 Korer J, Fitzsimmons JS. The effect of Huntington's chorea on family life. *Br J Soc Work.* 1985; **15**: 581–97.

66 Murdoch I. *The Sacred and Profane Love Machine.* London: Penguin; 1984.

67 Sheldon F. ABC of palliative care: bereavement. *BMJ.* 1998; **316**: 456–8.

68 Relf M, Machin L, Archer N. *Guidance for Bereavement Needs Assessment in Palliative Care*. London: Help the Hospices; 2008.

69 National Institute for Health and Clinical Excellence, op. cit.

70 Riches G, op. cit.

71 National Institute for Health and Clinical Excellence, op. cit.

72 Bruce EJ, op. cit.

73 National Institute for Health and Clinical Excellence, op. cit.

74 Parkes CM. A historical overview of the scientific study of bereavement. In: Stroebe MS, Hansson RO, Stroebe W, *et al.*, editors. *Handbook of Bereavement Research: consequences, coping and care*. Washington, DC: American Psychological Association; 2001. pp. 25–45.

75 Relf M, *et al.*, op. cit.

76 National Institute for Health and Clinical Excellence, op. cit.

77 Doyle D, Jeffrey D. *Palliative Care in the Home*. Oxford: Oxford University Press; 2000.

78 Joseph S, Linley PA. Growth following adversity: theoretical perspectives and implications for clinical practice. *Clin Psychol Rev.* 2006; 26(8): 1041–53.

79 Zisook S, op. cit.

80 Klass D, op. cit.

81 Nolen-Hoeksema SA, Larson J. *Coping with Loss*. New Jersey: Lawrence Erlbaum Associates; 1999.

82 Aubeeluck A (2005) *Developing a Scale to Measure the Impact of Huntington's Disease on the Quality of Life of Spousal Caregivers* [unpublished thesis]. University of Derby.

Conclusion

The contributions in this book help us to understand the offering that good palliative care can make to those who are either suffering from or caring for someone with a progressive long-term neurological condition (PLNTC).

Palliative care established itself as a clinical speciality in the 1980s with the recognition by the Royal College of Physicians of palliative medicine as a sub specialty of general medicine and it has been predominantly associated with the care of cancer patients since then. This book demonstrates the positive and life enhancing effect that the palliative approach to care can bring to those with PLTNCs.

Palliative care has not only been significant in dramatically improving the care of those with life limiting conditions but has also enabled the patient and family to be seen as a unit of care, each with interrelated needs for help, support and advice. Professionals responsible for referring patients for palliative care sometimes need help to recognise the constructive impact that this care can have on individuals and their families: this may help to ensure that those with PLTNC can access this expertise at appropriate times during their illness.

In this book we have sought to bring to attention and clarify some of the key issues and themes in the palliative care of people with PLTNCs and to provide indications of how these need to be acknowledged and addressed as part of an ongoing assessment process.

Central to palliative care and also referenced in the National Service Framework for Long-term (Neurological) Conditions is the need for a multidisciplinary approach to care, drawing on the skill and knowledge of all members of the multidisciplinary team. This runs in parallel with a holistic approach to care that embraces the needs of the whole person and those that care for them, incorporating the emotional, physical, spiritual, and social components of illness. Working with these principles of care in the field of neurological conditions depends on partnerships between those who specialise in palliative care and neurology teams, as well as good points of contact between these and the generalist staff who provide more regular support to the patient and family – the

GP and district nurse for example. There is real necessity for these partnerships to establish and to encourage the development of services in this country for people with PLTNCs to combine expertise and help identify the best time for referral to palliative care to be made. Working together to combine knowledge and skill is the best way of meeting the complex needs that patients and their families are likely to experience over time.

The book highlights the unpredictable and different trajectories that people living with PLTNCs can have and the requirement for these to be considered as part of the assessment process. It also identifies the need for best practice tools that have been developed with cancer patients in mind to be reviewed and revised to fit those with PLTNCs.

By its definition a progressive illness will not be cured, however the ability to help, support and have a significant effect for an individual is demonstrated through the application of the palliative approach to care. Curative care and palliative care exist side by side and at times the emphasis will shift and change, along with the need for professionals who are assessing the individual to respond and adapt to the changing situations. The model in Figure A illustrates how this can work in practice.

From the chapters in this book it is clear that the principles of palliative care that have been traditionally applied to people with cancer; the focus on quality of life; and team working and adherence to the framework of palliative care as defined by the World Health Organization are all acknowledged as being equally transferable to those people with PLTNCs. There is a requirement for palliative care to be seen as a key component for people with PLTNCs and their carers.

One of the profound influences on care is that death, which will come to all of us, does not need to be a negative experience but one that can improve

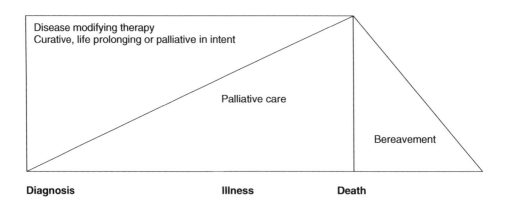

FIGURE A: Model for curative and palliative care
Source: *Cancer Control: knowledge into action: WHO guide for effective programmes; palliative care.* World Health Organization, Series 11; 2007.

family relationships and can help inner strengths to emerge, bringing a positive contribution to the end stage of someone's life. Both professional colleagues and carers should be greatly encouraged by the value that a palliative approach to care can bring to people with PLTNCs. Professionals, carers or patients can initiate a request for a referral to be made to a palliative care team for advice and support and this should be made at the first opportunity. The ability to control symptoms can maximise someone's quality of life and the ongoing assessment and sharing of expertise can be life changing for both the individual and family.

The effect and impact on the life of those who care for someone with a PLTNC can be profound; depending on the type of illness, care can be required for many years. Those years contain many peaks, troughs and periods of uncertainty. Through this time the caregivers become increasingly knowledgeable about the illness and the requirements of the person they have been caring for. Caregivers also experience loss and stress while taking care of their loved ones, therefore addressing the needs of caregivers is vital and we need to ensure that service provision is planned to help those people with PLTNCs and their carers to include timely access to palliative services, care and advice.

There is also a need for further research that draws on the expertise and experiences of those affected by PLTNCs to inform care giving in the future, care that can be tailored to those with PLTNCs. It is essential to maintain a balance between a social model of care focused on living with a disease and maintaining independence and not ignore or deny palliative needs.

Some people with PLTNCs lack capacity to make decisions, and this can be an area of care where needs do differ from that of cancer patients. Therefore advance care planning in these situations is required and staff need to be familiar with the specific processes related to the Mental Capacity Act 2005 to enable 'best interest' decisions to be made based on the law and sound ethical principles. This draws attention to the training required for professionals and carers and the need for continued investment in this area. Education is key to the dissemination of new knowledge and the development of new approaches and attitudes.

Good practice in palliative care is something that all disciplines and specialties need to embrace. Learning and skills need to be shared into wider settings where people with PLTNCs are cared for, to include both primary care and the care home sector. Professionals need to seize the day and work in partnership to create a responsive, helpful and cohesive team approach to palliative care to the benefit of both patients and carers.

This book helps us begin to learn, understand and appreciate the commonalities and differences between the model of care based on those with cancer and the model of care for people with PLTNCs and what these differences mean to the delivery of care.

Index